Practical Approaches To The Treatment Of Heart Failure

Practical Approaches To The Treatment Of Heart Failure

Roger M. Mills Jr., M.D.
Professor of Medicine
Clinical Director, Division of Cardiovascular Medicine
University of Kentucky College of Medicine
Lexington, Kentucky

James B. Young, M.D.
Head
Section of Heart Failure and Cardiac Transplant Medicine
Kaufman Center for Heart Failure
Department of Cardiology
The Cleveland Clinic Foundation
Cleveland, Ohio

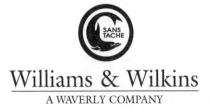

Williams & Wilkins
A WAVERLY COMPANY

BALTIMORE • PHILADELPHIA • LONDON • PARIS • BANGKOK
HONG KONG • MUNICH • SYDNEY • TOKYO • WROCLAW

Editor: Jonathan W. Pine, Jr.
Managing Editor: Leah Ann Kiehne Hayes
Marketing Manager: Daniell T. Griffin
Production Coordinator: Raymond E. Reter
Project Editor: Paula C. Williams
Designer: Artech, Baltimore, Maryland
Cover Designer: Artech, Baltimore, Maryland
Typesetter: TCSystems, Inc., Shippensburg, Pennsylvania
Printer & Binder: Vicks Lithograph & Printing Corporation, Yorkville, New York
Digitized Illustrations: TCSystems, Inc., Shippensburg, Pennsylvania

Printed in the United States of America

Library of Congress Cataloging-in-Publication Data

Practical approaches to the treatment of heart failure / editors,
  Roger M. Mills, Jr., James B. Young.
    p.   cm.
  Includes bibliographical references and index.
  ISBN 0-683-18104-1   1. Heart failure. I. Mills, Roger M. II. Young, James B.
  [DNLM: 1. Heart Failure, Congestive—therapy. 2. Heart Failure,
  Congestive—physiopathology. 3. Heart Failure, Congestive—
  diagnosis. WG 370 P895 1998]
  RC685.C53P73 1998
  616.1'29—dc21
  DNLM/DLC
  for Library of Congress   97-41999
                                    CIP

98 99 00 01 02
1 2 3 4 5 6 7 8 9 10

To my patients, colleagues, and trainees, who have taught me far more than I have taught them, and to my parents, who both succumbed to heart failure.

RMM

To my wife, Claire, my daughters Christine and Rebecca, and my sons James II and Joseph, who lovingly accepted many stolen moments.

JBY

Preface

Heart failure is epidemic. There is an estimated 3 to 4 million patients diagnosed as having heart failure in the United States presently and approximately 400,000 individuals develop symptomatic heart failure each year. These figures are likely underestimates, since they largely rely on the diagnosis of congestive heart failure, the tip of the iceberg. It is also disturbing to note that the incidence of heart failure more than doubles with each decade after the age of 45 and approximately 35% of heart failure patients are hospitalized each year. Heart failure is the only cardiovascular disease with increasing prevalence, and it is the leading and most expensive cause of hospitalization in patients after age 65. The average length of hospital stay for heart failure is 9.1 days, with an average cost of $12,049. Primary care physicians treat the vast majority of these people, predominantly in outpatient settings. Despite rather dramatic improvements in our ability to care for the sickest of these patients in highly specialized clinics, available data suggest that most patients do not currently receive state-of-the-art therapy.

We intend this book to serve as a pragmatic guide to the most contemporary concepts of diagnosis and treatment of heart failure. It is meant to be a working guidebook that belongs in the clinic rather than in the office or reference library. Our approach includes the presentation of physiologic principles, allowing for a better understanding of the rationale of therapeutic suggestions. We hope this will clarify those aspects of heart failure patient care that seem counterintuitive. Only critical references are included. Most chapters conclude with a summary that reinforces the relevance of the chapter contents to patient care. Numerous tables, flow charts, and clinical treatment algorithms are included to make quick reference to difficult questions simple. For professionals looking for a critical care pathway approach to the patient with heart failure, the text provides documentation of current standards of care.

Initially, we each envisioned a single-author textbook. The complexity of the task, as well as an enjoyable collaborative relationship, convinced us that working together would be productive. We have tried to maintain uniformity of both prose style, and approach. It should be emphasized that this text represents *our* approach, not the only approach, to diagnosing and treating heart failure patients. Consistency, however, is critical to quality, and quality is a major issue.

We hope that this volume serves as an accessible, friendly consultant, offering the insights gleaned from our highly specialized heart failure practices to physicians and other health care professionals facing practical problems with their own patients.

Contributors

Randy W. Braith, Ph.D.
Assistant Professor
College of Health and Human
Performance
Center for Exercise Science
University of Florida
Gainesville, Florida

Jamie Beth Conti, M.D.
Assistant Professor
Division of Cardiology
University of Florida
Gainesville, Florida

Andrew M. Cross Jr., M.D.
Assistant Professor
Division of Cardiovascular
Medicine
University of Kentucky College of
Medicine
Lexington, Kentucky

Anne B. Curtis, M.D.
Associate Professor
Director of Clinical
Electrophysiology
Division of Cardiology
University of Florida
Gainesville, Florida

**Eileen Handberg, A.R.N.P.,
M.S.N.**
Assistant Director of Clinical
Programs
Division of Cardiology

University of Florida College of
Medicine
Gainesville, Florida

Patrick M. McCarthy, M.D.
Department of Thoracic and
Cardiovascular Surgery
Kaufman Center for Heart Failure
The Cleveland Clinic Foundation
Cleveland, Ohio

Santosh G. Menon, M.D.
Assistant Professor
Medical Director, Heart
Transplant Program
Division of Cardiovascular
Medicine
University of Kentucky, College of
Medicine
Lexington, Kentucky

Roger M. Mills Jr., M.D.
Professor of Medicine
Clinical Director, Division of
Cardiovascular Medicine
University of Kentucky College of
Medicine
Lexington, Kentucky

Nicholas G. Smedira, M.D.
Department of Thoracic and
Cardiovascular Surgery
Kaufman Center for Heart Failure
The Cleveland Clinic Foundation
Cleveland, Ohio

Sharen Thompson, L.C.S.W.
Department of Social Services
Shands Hospital at the University
of Florida
Gainesville, Florida

Michael A. Welsch, Ph.D.
Assistant Professor
Louisiana State University
Baton Rouge, Louisiana

**Margaret Kay Worley, A.R.N.P.,
M.N., C.C.R.N.**
Clinical Trials Director
Division of Cardiovascular
Medicine
University of Kentucky College of
Medicine
Lexington, Kentucky

James B. Young, M.D.
Head
Section of Heart Failure and
Cardiac Transplant Medicine
Kaufman Center for Heart Failure
Department of Cardiology
The Cleveland Clinic Foundation
Cleveland, Ohio

Contents

Section 1

Background and Current Concepts

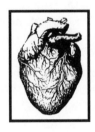

Chapter 1

The Heart Failure Syndrome
Historic Perceptions, Contemporary Definition, and Diagnosis

James B. Young

Heart failure is now pandemic (1). It is extremely important, therefore, to focus a great deal of attention on this difficulty if we expect to see a significant decrement in morbidity and mortality. Despite the decreasing mortality rates from coronary heart disease and stroke in the United States, the incidences of heart failure and related hospitalizations are increasing dramatically and rapidly. Table 1.1 summarizes why we should shift attention to this malady.

The number of patients in the United States with congestive heart failure—a small subset of the overall heart failure population—is approximately 4 million; 15 million patients worldwide are affected by congestive heart failure. Congestive heart failure is the only cardiovascular difficulty believed to have an increasing prevalence; its incidence doubles in the general population with each decade over age 45. Indeed, it is thought that more than half of the symptomatic heart failure patients are over age 65, and the prevalence of the syndrome increases with age. Because the U.S. population is aging and the prevalence of symptomatic heart failure rises with age, we can expect almost 6 million symptomatic congestive heart failure patients in 2030.

Mortality is high in this syndrome; males generally have a 50% chance of death within 24 months after the appearance of overt congestive symptoms. Heart failure is the third leading cause of hospitalization for all patients in the United States and the principal cause in individuals over 65 years old. Heart failure represents the largest and most expensive diagnosis-related group (DRG) receiving reimbursement from the Health Care Financing Administration (HCFA). The 3-month readmission rate after an index hospitalization for heart failure is 20–50%; well more than 33% of all patients who have been diagnosed with congestive heart failure are hospitalized annually.

Table 1.1.   Why Focus on Heart Failure?

- In the United States, 4 million people have symptomatic heart failure.
- Worldwide, 15 million patients are affected.
- In 1990, 700,000 hospital discharges were patients with a primary diagnosis of heart failure (four times the number from 1971).
- In 1990, 280,000 deaths were caused primarily by heart failure.
- Half of all heart failure patients are 65+ years old (incidence increases from 3/1000 males aged 50–59 to 27/1000 males aged 80–89).
- Because the U.S. population is aging, the prevalence of heart failure is expected to rise and is estimated to be almost 6 million by 2030.
- The overall mortality in symptomatic males is 50% at 24 months.
- Congestive heart failure is the largest and most expensive DRG in the United States.
- Direct annual expenditures for heart failure have been estimated to be $10–40 billion (in 1994, HCFA alone spent $545 billion for congestive heart failure).
- Each heart failure patient's hospitalization costs $6,000–12,000.
- The 3-month readmission rate is 20–50%.
- Heart failure pathophysiology and studies in molecular biodynamics are providing new insights.
- The definition of heart failure is changing.
- The focus is shifting to early identification of patients at risk and to prevention programs.
- Clinical trial data are available to help the clinician design evidence-based treatment paradigms.
- Symptomatic heart failure patients are now commonly prescribed multiple pharmaceuticals.
- Managing heart failure patients requires careful consideration of surgical and medical options.

DRG, diagnosis-related group; *HCFA,* Health Care Financing Administration.

Fortunately, insights into the pathophysiologic process of heart failure and, in particular, molecular biodynamics are growing (2). New findings have prompted the reconsideration of the definition of *heart failure;* and, as will be discussed, the syndrome is actually much more broad and inclusive than the term *congestive heart failure* implies (3–6). A more appropriate definition of this syndrome allows us to focus on the early identification of individuals at risk for developing symptomatic heart failure, before they exhibit overtly perturbed cardiocirculatory dynamics (7–9). This approach emphasizes the institution of prevention programs (9). Indeed, clinical trial data from the 1980s and 1990s have made it possible for us to design specific evidence-based treatment paradigms that can clearly reduce the morbidity and mortality of the heart failure syndrome. The challenge is great; despite the advances made in the attenuation of morbidity and mortality of heart failure, we have fallen short of the optimal mark. The difficulty is still tremendously problematic. It is important to review the evolution of insight that prompted the aggressive contemporary management of patients with heart failure. To consider optimal present-day management paradigms for these patients, we must establish a well-reasoned definition of heart failure that sets contemporary insight into the context of historic perspective. This allows us to make rational recommendations regarding the various therapies available that are designed to interdict pathophysiologic heart failure, lessening the morbidity and high mortality that invariably accompanies the syndrome. The socioeconomic benefits of providing better care for heart failure patients are obvious.

HISTORIC PERSPECTIVES OF HEART FAILURE

The clinical syndrome of heart failure has been recognized and treated for hundreds, perhaps thousands, of years (10). Table 1.2 lists the progress of insight in an historical context, emphasizing that early concern arose with edematous conditions. Although the intricate interrelationship of the heart and the peripheral cardiovascular system has only recently been defined, reference to dropsical conditions likely caused by cardiac decompensation can be found in the literature of ancient civilizations.

Though there is little surviving evidence to suggest that cardiovascular disease was present in early human populations, ancient Egyptian writing and the contemporary study of mummified cadavers

Table 1.2.   Historic Perceptions of Heart Failure

- Heart failure is a dropsical condition.
- Heart failure is caused by a central pump inadequacy.
- Heart failure is caused by decompensated ventricular hypertrophy.
- Heart failure is a dysfunction of the circulatory system.
- Heart failure is an endocrinopathy.
- Heart failure is a fever.
- Heart failure is a complicated milieu of pump dysfunction, myocardial remodeling, humoral perturbation, and subsequent circulatory insufficiency.

suggest that Egyptians had a rudimentary understanding of the pulse and heartbeat and that cardiovascular disease was present. Although ancient Greek cognoscenti likely focused specifically on cardiovascular pulse assessment, linking deviations to disease, Egyptian physicians seemingly were aware of the cardiovascular system and, possibly, its relationship to disease. Morley-Davies and Nolan (10) recently suggested that an initial clinical description of the heart failure syndrome exists in the Ebers Papyrus, dating from 1600 B.C. (about three centuries before Moses).

When studying historic documents and tracing historic commentary concerning heart failure, we have the problem of trying to relate dropsical or fluid retention states directly to cardiovascular illness. Dropsy can be caused by many noncardiac pathologic conditions, including renal, hepatic, and endocrine disorders, which, even today, are challenging to diagnose and separate from primary cardiovascular conditions. Nevertheless, one of the more dramatic allusions to heart failure in ancient times may be Luke's description of Jesus curing a dropsical patient (Luke 14:2–4).

To more specifically link cardiac and cardiovascular dysfunction to the development of a heart failure syndrome, appreciation of the relationship of the heart, functioning as a synchronized central pump, to the peripheral circulation, providing systemic organ perfusion, was necessary. Ancient Egyptians, Greeks, and Romans struggled with rudimentary knowledge of the pulse; but it was not until the Italian Renaissance that Realdo Colombo (1516–1559) and Girolamo Fabrizio d'Acquapendente (1533–1619) set the stage for William Harvey (1578–1657) to conceive of and describe circulation of blood (11). Their observations were based on seminal publications by Andreus Vesalius (1514–1564), a professor of anatomy at the University of Padua, who published the first great anatomic work. It is notable that Vesalius could not demonstrate the intraventricular pores that Galen (131–201) had suggested were responsible for circulating blood from the right side of the circulation to the left.

Although Harvey's work, which detailed the anatomic nuances of blood circulation, was not published until 1628 (the year Shakespeare died), what is likely the first well-characterized description of congestive heart failure appeared in the Middle Ages. In a biography of her father, Byzantine emperor Alexius I (r. 1081–1118), Anna Comnena wrote that he suffered from an illness characterized by an irregular pulse and associated with dyspnea, which forced him to "sit upright to breath at all" (12).

Several descriptions of congestive heart failure appeared after the publication of Harvey's work. Bartoletti (1576–1630) related case histories of patients with a peculiar dyspnea after which sudden death was often noted. He described patients who had suffered for significant periods from respiratory difficulties prompted by walking, which was relieved with rest, and characterized by suffocation.

As scientific knowledge evolved in the seventeenth century and detailed descriptions of cardiac pathologic states (e.g., valvular heart disease) appeared, it became evident that cardiac abnormalities could be responsible for fluid retention, or dropsy. Hermann Boerhaave (1668–1738) is generally credited with being the first to link anasarca to cardiac dysfunction; but Morely-Davies and Nolan (10) suggest that the first more contemporaneous definition of heart failure actually appeared in Richard Lower's *Tractatus de Cordis* (1669):

> *But when the parenchyma of the heart has been harmed by various diseases its motion is necessarily much altered; for if the parenchyma of the heart is burdened with too much fat, labors under inflammation, abscess or wound, so that it cannot vibrate or contract without great trouble or difficulty, it soon gives up its motion, the movement of the blood, also to the same degree, becomes weak and languid.*

Constrictive pericardial disease and pericardial effusion that causes cardiac tamponade are also elegantly described in this seminal text.

In 1685, a century before William Withering published his marvelously accurate monograph on the Shropshire maid's remedy for dropsy, Thomas Sydenham (13) suggested bleeding, purges, vomiting, blistering, garlic, and wine or good ale as dropsical therapies. It is interesting that these therapies persisted in many reports, in one fashion or another, through to the twentieth century.

It was Withering's seminal publication in 1785 that so elegantly described the use of foxglove tea, which contained the now well known cardiac glycoside digitalis, to ameliorate select dropsical conditions (14). Withering knew the implications of giving foxglove tea to the wrong patients or in improper dosages. In fact, he vehemently objected to prescribing foxglove to dropsical patients with robust and regular pulse, noting that these individuals simply became toxic and did not exhibit diuresis. Withering also pointed out that highly concentrated foxglove tea or excessive administration could precipitate a disturbing spectrum of nausea, vomiting, visual disturbance, and cardiovascular collapse, which we now know are symptoms of digitalis toxicity.

A careful review of Withering's writings reveals that patients who responded to his therapy likely had dropsical conditions rooted in cardiovascular abnormalities associated with atrial fibrillation. Indeed, Withering nicely characterized the weak and thready pulse coupled with pale continence that characterized dropsical patients he thought would respond to the herbal preparation. Dropsical patients with nephrotic syndrome, tuberculous peritonitis, myxedema, or cirrhosis of the liver—common conditions in the late eighteenth century—would, of course, be more likely to have robust and regular pulses with ruddy complexion and, therefore, would not be expected to experience diuresis with the foxglove herbal preparation. Withering's observations and lessons hold true today.

We should remember several important tenets of heart failure therapeutics that emphasize the necessity of ensuring that any given patient's symptoms and physical findings are, in fact, caused by heart failure and not some other disease that can also produce a dropsical condition. Furthermore, using the most appropriate medications, generally those defined as effective and safe in clinical trials or in carefully conducted bias-controlled protocols, is essential to success.

Protocols for treating dropsical conditions caused by heart failure evolved slowly, despite increased insight into the relationship of the heart to the condition. Jean Nicolas, baron de Corvisart-Desmarets, in 1812, continued to suggest purges, bleeding, leeches, squill (a cardiac glycoside preparation), physical removal of ascites and pleural effusions, puncture of edematous legs, and nitrated drinks (15). More aggressive use of diuretics, although most preparations were toxic and weak, occurred in the mid-nineteenth century; prescriptions consisted of mercurial preparations (largely calomel) and potassium bitartrate. Subcutaneous morphine sulfate injections were used in the 1860s to ameliorate dyspnea; and the Karrell diet, which was primarily low-sodium skim milk, was proposed in 1866.

Austin Flint, in 1873, suggested digitalis, ether, dry cupping, opiates, cathartics, incisions, and organ cavity space puncture to relieve dropsy caused by decompensated ventricular hypertrophy (16). Flint was the first to suggest that the heart went through a long period of quiescent compensated hypertrophy in settings of valvular insufficiency or stenosis, before decompensating and leading to a congestive heart failure syndrome. He may have been the first to have actually used the term *heart failure* in the modern context.

Southey tubes, which were inserted into leg lymphatics to treat edema, were introduced in 1877; and bromides for sedation were also frequently used during this time. Rudimentary diuretics in the late nineteenth century included theophylline, theobromine, and urea salts. Catharsis and bloodletting through venesection were common treatments at the turn of the century as well.

Supplemental oxygen was used in the early 1900s; and in 1910, James MacKenzie suggested that amyl nitrate was useful, as was digitalis, oxygen, purgatives, and venesection (12). Mercurial diuretics were used with increasing frequency in the 1920s and 1930s; and during this period, thyroidectomy was employed to treat more severe cases of congestive heart failure. The cardiac chair was introduced about this time, and diet therapies began to focus seriously on water and salt restriction. Bed rest was virtually always a component of congestive heart failure therapies prescribed through the first half of the twentieth century, culminating in the 1960s with Burch's recommendation of complete and compulsive long-term bed rest when cardiomyopathy was diagnosed.

In 1937, Fishberg recommended that atrial fibrillation and flutter associated with congestive heart failure be treated with quinidine and digitalis (17). The carbonic anhydrase inhibitor acetazolemide was introduced in 1950; and hexamethonium, the potent α-blocking antihypertensive agent, appeared in 1956. Ligation of the inferior vena cava was a treatment used in 1952; and thyroidectomy or radioactive iodine ablation of the thyroid gland for severe heart failure was proposed as late as 1956 (18).

Intra-aortic balloon counterpulsation for hemodynamic collapse secondary to severe heart failure was first proposed in 1961; surgical treatment of left ventricular aneurysm was attempted in 1962. In the 1960s, the future Nobel Peace Prize laureate Bernard Lown promoted electrical cardioversion for atrial fibrillation complicating heart failure, and this was the era in which cardiac valvular surgery as treatment for heart failure caused by valvular stenosis or insufficiency began in earnest. Thiazide diuretics were introduced in 1962, furosemide in 1965, and ethacrynic acid in 1966. The first human-to-human cardiac transplant was performed in 1967.

The modern paradigm shift in the treatment of heart failure occurred in the 1970s, when use of vasodilating drugs began; earlier treatments had been rooted in cardiac glycoside prescription and diuretic therapies. New inotropic preparations were pursued, and dopamine was introduced in 1972 and dobutamine in 1975. Nitroprusside became available in 1974, and hydralazine in 1977. Hurst et al. (19), recommended that patients decrease physical and emotional stress; follow a low-salt diet; and take digitalis, diuretics (thiazide, furosemide, ethacrynic acid, spironolactone, and mercurial agents), and vasodilators (nitroprusside, isosorbide dinitrate, and hydralazine) in certain circumstances.

The decade of the 1980s is best described as the era of angiotensin-converting enzyme inhibitor therapy. The focus on agents that block neurohormonal perturbations characteristic of heart failure is counterintuitive but is supported by many landmark clinical trials performed in the late 1970s. New drugs at this time included captopril (1980) and enalapril (1984). The last two decades have seen the continued evolution of heart failure treatment and better, but still incomplete, clarification of the role of digitalis and β-blockers in heart failure patients. Furthermore, clinical practices that appear intuitively logical in heart setting were proved to be detrimental when tested by formal clinical trials. For example, several inotropic agents with various degrees of vasodilating properties that seemed to improve heart failure symptoms were actually associated with higher mortality rates. Because heart failure patients frequently die of malignant ventricular arrhythmias, it seemed logical to suppress the dysrhythmias; unfortunately, some antiarrhythmics were found to be deleterious in the face of left ventricular dysfunction. Other trials suggested that calcium channel blockers, although potent arteriolar dilators, often produce more problems than benefits in heart failure cohorts.

Today there is an increased professional and public awareness of the heart failure epidemic, and new diagnosis and treatment strategies have developed that focus on the asymptomatic patient with left ventricular dysfunction. Indeed, an understanding has emerged that heart failure is not solely a congested condition but rather a complicated spectrum of cardiac dysfunction that can be seen in patients who are entirely asymptomatic, as well as in those manifesting pulmonary edema or cardiogenic shock.

As we enter the twenty-first century, another paradigm shift in heart failure treatment is occurring; the focus is now on the interdiction of the α- and β-adrenergic cascades, known to be important in heart failure, and of the recently identified inflammatory components of the syndrome. Indeed, although β-blockers were first given to heart failure patients in the 1970s, two decades of drug package inserts admonish their use in this setting. Recent experience seems to suggest that more complete blockade of the renin–angiotensin–aldosterone pathways in conjunction with α- and β-adrenergic blockade represents a beneficial strategy in these patients.

The 1990s have also been marked by a dramatic rise in the use of mechanical left ventricular assist devices, which have been demonstrated to be life-saving options in seriously ill patients with cardiogenic shock. These remarkable machines have frequently been used to bridge patients to cardiac transplantation and, even more recently, to recovery, with subsequent removal of the devices. Programs have begun to evaluate the use of assist devices as long-term treatment options for advanced heart failure as an alternative to cardiac transplantation.

A CONTEMPORARY DEFINITION OF HEART FAILURE

Heart failure has for some time been viewed as a situation in which the contractile apparatus, or structural integrity of the heart, cannot pump blood adequately, causing a decrement in stroke volume with a subsequent alteration in peripheral bed perfusion (20,21). Often, the earliest manifestations of heart failure are subtle and escape our ability to quantitate significant changes. In the past, heart failure was generally associated with increased venous pressure and dropsical conditions. This definition focused on late-stage clinical settings with overt, obvious symptoms and physical findings that are generally related to a combination of volume overload and markedly reduced forward cardiac output. Now that we understand better the pathophysiologic process of myocardial and circulatory failure, a definition based on more contemporaneous insight is required (Table 1.3).

We know that heart failure is a milieu or syndrome characterized by the perturbation of multiple neuroendocrine, humoral, and inflammatory feedback loops that develop after some sort of myocardial injury causes hemodynamic changes; the changes can be extraordinarily subtle. In fact, initial homeostatic cardiovascular compensation can be quite effective, and symptoms and physical findings traditionally associated with congestive heart failure are often not detectable during the earliest stages of heart failure. Nevertheless, heart failure is, indeed, present and manifest by abnormal molecular biodynamic events that result, ultimately, in ventricular hypertrophy and cardiac dilatation, hallmarks of the so-called cardiac remodeling.

As the compensatory mechanisms themselves become problematic (many actually exacerbate the detrimental remodeling process), symptoms and physical findings (again, generally related to congestion or low cardiac output) develop. Clinicians have, therefore, moved toward a more encompassing definition of heart failure, one that highlights abnormalities noted at the physiologic, hormonal,

Table 1.3.   Creating a Contemporary Definition of Heart Failure

- Myocardial injury causes acute or chronic myocyte dysfunction (systolic and/or diastolic).
- Myocyte passive tension and workloads change.
- Myocyte interstitial matrix stiffens.
- Peripheral vascular bed blood flow is altered (generally decreased in a subtle fashion).
- Subsequent mechanical, humoral, neurohormonal, and inflammatory responses appear in an attempt to create systemic organ flow compensation.
- Compensatory mechanisms ultimately produce a maladaptive circulatory state that is characterized by myocyte hypertrophy and cardiac dilatation (the components of remodeling).
- Patients may present without symptoms or suffer from a variety of fatigue, dyspnea, or dropsical states that fluctuate in severity based on treatment protocols, diet, physical conditioning, and diseases precipitating the heart failure syndrome.

cellular, subcellular organelle, and genetic levels long before hemo-dynamic alterations traditionally associated with congestive heart failure can be seen. It is important to stress the fact that heart failure should not be defined solely as a congestive state or congestive heart failure but, rather, should include a broad spectrum of adjectives, such as acute or chronic, right sided or left sided, systolic or diastolic (Table 1.3). In the future, as insight into the syndrome's pathophysio-logic processes grows, additional adjectives will be included that more precisely describe each individual patient. It is likely that these adjectives will refer to many specific hormonal, humoral, or in-flammatory aberrations that characterize various stages of the syn-drome.

When creating a contemporary definition of heart failure, one should start with the understanding that myocardial injury causes acute or chronic myocyte dysfunction (systolic and/or diastolic), lead-ing to a change in regional myocyte passive tension and workload (Chapter 2). As systolic and diastolic ventricular functions become impaired, the myocyte interstitial matrix stiffens. Mechanical abnor-malities develop such that stroke volume is decreased and blood flow to the peripheral vascular bed is altered. Initially, flows are subtly decreased in the majority of cases. Subsequent mechanical, humoral, neurohormonal, and inflammatory responses develop in an attempt to maintain systemic organ flow compensation and initi-ate the reparative or healing processes (Chapter 3). These compensa-tory mechanisms themselves ultimately produce a maladaptive circu-latory state, which sets the stage for perpetuating the heart failure syndrome. Syndrome perpetuation is characterized by remodeling (left ventricular hypertrophy and dilation) of various degrees. Pa-tients may be asymptomatic or suffer from several symptoms, which differ in severity based on treatment protocols, other diseases, and lifestyle choices.

Using this definition, not only can we ameliorate symptoms with tailored treatment strategies but, by identifying early patients with insidious hemodynamic and hormonal perturbation, we can also attenuate heart failure morbidity and decrease mortality with thera-peutic measures. Indeed, in an epidemiologic sense, it is more im-portant to treat patients with asymptomatic left ventricular dysfunc-tion than those with symptomatic heart failure.

COUPLING THE DEFINITION OF HEART FAILURE TO A DIAGNOSIS

It should be obvious that to treat heart failure patients properly, an appropriate diagnosis must be made (Table 1.4). Diagnosing heart failure no longer simply consists of auscultating pulmonary rales and a gallop rhythm in patients with pedal edema or dyspnea. Individuals will have a wide spectrum of symptoms, which include a characteristic predominance of systolic or diastolic dysfunction, and selective cardiac chamber enlargement (atrial versus ventricular and right sided versus left sided) coupled to structural integrity of the cardiac valves. Diagnostic evaluations must consider the various diseases that precipitate abnormal chamber filling or emptying. Efforts must be made, therefore, to determine the cause of cardiac failure, stage its severity (particularly attempting to identify patients with early and nonedematous states), and identify factors that may have precipitated clinical decompensation (usually manifest by volume overload).

It is, however, extremely important to remember that not all dropsical individuals have heart failure and that complaints of dyspnea should not automatically point to cardiac failure. Ask the following critical questions whenever heart failure is considered as a diagnosis: *(a)* Is myocardial or circulatory failure actually present? *(b)* What caused the problem? *(c)* What is the patient's prognosis? *(d)* Can the symptoms be eliminated or ameliorated? *(e)* What can be done to cure or treat the underlying difficulty? *(f)* Can the progression of the syndrome be halted?

Table 1.4.   Diagnosing Heart Failure

- Recognize the syndrome: not everyone with rales and edema has heart failure.
- Determine the cause of the syndrome: coronary obstruction with active ischemia can be ameliorated.
- Clarify the factors precipitating congestion: salt restriction and afterload reduction are critical.
- Stage the severity of the syndrome: polypharmacy may not be necessary for asymptomatic left ventricular dysfunction.
- Tailor the therapy to pathophysiologic observation: relief of congestive symptoms may require multiple diuretic classes.

As might be gathered from the contemporary definition, evaluations should be planned that allow specific tailoring of appropriate therapeutic maneuvers believed likely to prevent, cure, or treat various aspects of the heart failure syndrome. The early identification of patients with asymptomatic ventricular dysfunction but no substantive symptoms is essential if we are to optimize the likelihood of preventing further myocardial dysfunction and clinical deterioration. Indeed, this definition of heart failure, allows us to consider specifically the left ventricular systolic dysfunction that frequently accompanies hypertension or coronary artery disease states.

The Agency for Health Care Policy and Research (AHCPR) recently published guidelines for evaluating and treating heart failure patients (22). Its diagnostic algorithm is, however, focused on symptomatic patients with stable, generally compensated congestive heart failure not requiring hospitalization. The algorithm, though somewhat narrow, is still quite reasonable. It suggests specific and objective evaluation of all patients with complaints that could possibly be related to congestive heart failure, such as paroxysmal nocturnal dyspnea, orthopnea, dyspnea on exertion, lower extremity edema, decreased exercise tolerance, unexplained confusion, altered mental status, nonspecific fatigue (in the elderly), and gastrointestinal or abdominal symptoms that might relate to mesenteric congestion (such as nausea, abdominal pain, bloating, and ascites).

Important physical examination findings should include data that suggest increased central vascular volume, such as elevated jugular venous pressure, positive abdominal jugular reflex, a third heart sound, a laterally displaced apical cardiac impulse, pulmonary rales not clearing with cough, and peripheral edema not caused by simple venous insufficiency. Patients with suspected congestive heart failure should then have their left ventricular function evaluated (echocardiographic and radionuclide scintigraphic studies are choices) so that the degree of systolic left ventricular dysfunction can be determined. Echocardiography is believed to be more advantageous than radionuclide scintigraphy because it permits concomitant assessment of valvular heart disease, ventricular hypertrophy, and cardiac chamber dimension. Furthermore, this technique is generally less expensive and more readily available than is radionuclide ventriculography. Ancillary studies include an electrocardiogram, a complete blood count, urinalysis, serum creatinine and serum albumin tests, and a thyroid function test.

These recommendations can be modified to encompass a broader scope of individuals with asymptomatic left ventricular dysfunction (and, therefore, heart failure) by including patients at high risk for occult left systolic ventricular dysfunction or left ventricular hypertrophy. It is prudent to perform echocardiography in every patient who is suffering from or has had an acute myocardial infarction. In addition, elderly patients with chronic hypertension or who have had coronary artery bypass graft surgery or percutaneous coronary interventions for coronary artery disease (particularly in the setting of comorbid conditions, such as diabetes mellitus, cerebral vascular accidents, and peripheral vascular disease) should have echocardiography performed at some intermittent screening interval that has yet to be optimally defined.

It should be re-emphasized that this approach is quite different from earlier methods of diagnosing heart failure, which relied primarily on relating complaints of dyspnea, orthopnea, paroxysmal nocturnal dyspnea, and history of edema to physical findings of tachycardia, pulmonary rales, third heart sound, jugular venous distension, and pitting pedal edema. Table 1.5 summarizes the diagnostic criteria used in the Framingham Heart Study (23), the Study of Men Born in 1913 (24), and the Boston Heart Failure Scale (25), which all used, to a greater or lesser extent, these classic heart failure symptoms and signs. Certainly, patients with these complaints and findings will often have congestive heart failure, but these signs entirely miss the even larger cohort of heart failure patients with asymptomatic or minimally symptomatic ventricular dysfunction who are euvolemic. Indeed, the positive predictive value of paroxysmal nocturnal dyspnea, orthopnea, and history of edema with respect to a correct diagnosis of heart failure was only 26, 2, and 22%, respectively. Only the presence of a third heart sound had a positive predictive value greater than 50% (but still just 61%) with respect to physical findings correlating to a diagnosis of heart failure.

By using our operational definition of heart failure, we can better couple proposed treatments to insights gained from clinical trials regarding heart failure therapies (Chapter 4) and, after better understanding the implications of the cardiac (Chapter 2) and circulatory responses (Chapter 3) to injury, enter into treatment of these patients.

Table 1.5. Criteria Used for Diagnosis of Congestive Heart Failure in Clinical Studies

The Framingham Heart Study	The Study of Men Born in 1913	The Boston Scale Criteria
Major criteria • Paroxysmal nocturnal dyspnea • Neck vein distension • Rales • Cardiomegaly • Acute pulmonary edema • S3 gallop • Increased venous pressure (> 16 cm) • Circulation time ≥ 25 s • Hepatojugular reflux positive Minor criteria • Ankle edema • Night cough • Hepatomegaly • Pleural effusion • Vital capacity reduced by one-third from predicted • Tachycardia (≥ 120) Major or minor criterion • Weight loss of more than 4.5 kg over 5 days in response to treatment Definite CHF • Two major criteria or one major and two minor criteria	Cardiac scores • Heart disease history (0 = absent; 1 = past; 2 = past year) • Angina pectoris (0 = absent; 1 = past; 2 = past year) • Swollen legs evenings (0 = absent; 1 = present) • Dyspnea at night (0 = absent; 1 = present) • Rales (0 = absent; 1 = present) • Atrial fibrillation (0 = absent; 1 = present) Pulmonary scores • Bronchitis/asthma history (0 = absent; 1 = past; 2 = past year) • Cough, phlegm, wheezing (0 = absent; 1 = present) • Rhonchi (0 = absent; 2 = present) Stages of CHF 1: Cardiac scores only (higher = worse) 2: Cardiac score and dyspnea or cardiac score and treatment for CHF (higher = worse) 3: Cardiac score, dyspnea, and treatment for CHF (higher = worse) 4: Decreased with or because of CHF Latent CHF • Stage 1 Manifest CHF • Stages 2 and 3 (or 4)	Category I: History • Rest dyspnea (4 points) • Orthopnea (4 points) • Paroxysmal nocturnal dyspnea (3 points) • Dyspnea walking level (2 points) • Dyspnea climbing (1 point) Category II: physical examination • Heart rate: 91–110 (1 point); > 110 (2 points) • Jugular venous pressure elevation: > 6 cm H_2O (2 points); > 6 cm H_2O plus hepatomegaly or leg edema (3 points) • Lung rales: Basilar (1 point); more than basilar (2 points) • Wheezing (3 points) • Third heart sound (3 points) Category III: chest radiography • Alveolar pulmonary edema (4 points) • Interstitial pulmonary edema (3 points) • Bilateral pleural effusion (3 points) • Cardiothoracic ratio ≥ 0.50 (3 points) • Upper zone flow redistribution (2 points) Determine score • Point value within parentheses and no more than 4 points from each category allowed. The maximum possible is 12 points. Definite CHF • 8–12 points Possible CHF • 5–7 points

CHF, congestive heart failure.

REFERENCES
1. Starling RC. Health care impact of heart failure. In: Topol EJ. Textbook of cardiovascular medicine. Philadelphia: Lippincott, in press.
2. Young JB, Pratt CM. Hemodynamic and hormonal alterations in patients with heart failure: toward a contemporary definition of heart failure. Semin Nephrol 1994;14:427–440.
3. Young JB. Assessment of heart failure. In: Colucci WS, Braunwald E, eds., Atlas of heart diseases. Heart failure: cardiac function and dysfunction. St. Louis: Mosby, 1994.
4. Young JB, Farmer JA. The diagnostic evaluation of patients with heart failure. New York: Springer-Verlag, 1994.
5. Young JB. Contemporary management of patients with heart failure. Med Clin North Am 1995;79:1171–1192.
6. Young JB. Overview of medical therapy in heart failure: the challenge of rational polypharmacy. In: Balady GJ, Pina IL, eds., Exercise and heart failure. New York: Futura, 1997.
7. Armstrong PW, Moe CW. Medical advances in the treatment of congestive heart failure. Circulation 1993;88:2941–2952.
8. Chatterjee K. Heart failure therapy in evolution. Circulation 1996;94:2689–2693.
9. Cohn JN. The management of chronic heart failure. N Engl J Med 1996; 335:490–498.
10. Morley-Davies A, Nolan J. Heart failure: a historical context. In: McMurray JJV, Cleland JGF, eds., Heart failure in clinical practice. New York: Mosby, 1996.
11. Thiene G. The discovery of circulation and the origin of modern medicine during the Italian Renaissance. Cardiovasc Pathol 1997;6:79–88.
12. MacKenzie J. Diseases of the heart. London: n.p., 1910.
13. Sydenham T. A treatise of the gout and dropsy. In: The works of Thomas Sydenham, M.D.: On acute and chronic diseases. Vol. 2. London: Robinson, Otridge, Hayes, & Newbery, 1683.
14. Withering W. An account of the foxglove, and some of its medical uses: with practical remarks on dropsy and other diseases. London: Robinson & Paternoster-Row, 1785.
15. Corvisart-Desmarets JN. Essay on the organic diseases of the heart. Paris: n.p., 1812.
16. Flint A. A treatise on the principles and practice of medicine. 4th ed. Philadelphia: Lea, 1983.
17. Fishberg A. Heart disease. Philadelphia: Lea & Febiger, 1937.
18. Friedberg CK. Diseases of the heart. 2nd ed. Philadelphia: Saunders, 1956.
19. Hurst JW, Logue RJ, Schlant RC, Wenger NC., eds. The heart, arteries and veins. 4th ed. New York: McGraw-Hill, 1978.
20. Harris P. The problem of defining heart failure. Cardiovasc Drugs Ther 1994;8:447–452.
21. Dargie HJ. What is heart failure? In: McMurray JJV, Cleland JGF, eds., Heart failure in clinical practice. St. Louis: Mosby, 1996.
22. Konstam MA, Dracup K, Baker DW, et al. Heart failure: evaluation and care of patients with left-ventricular systolic dysfunction [Clinical practice guideline; AHCPR publication 94-0612]. Rockville, MD: Agency for Health Care Policy and Research, June 1994.
23. McKee PA, Castelli WP, McNamarra PM, et al. The natural history of congestive heart failure: the Framingham study. N Engl J Med 1971;285:1441–1446.
24. Eriksson H, Svardsudd K, Larsson B, et al. Risk factors for heart failure in the general population. The study of men born in 1913. Eur Heart J 1989;10:647–656.
25. Remes J, Miettenen H, Reunanen A, Pyorala K. Validity of clinical diagnosis of heart failure in primary health care. Eur Heart J 1991;12:315–321.

Chapter 2

The Cardiac Response to Injury

James B. Young

The root problem of heart failure is some form of cardiac injury that leads to disruption of normal myocyte cellular homeostasis, structural abnormality, or both. Failure to maintain normal cardiovascular homeostasis is the essence of today's definition of heart failure. Disruption of the system occurs at both the macroscopic circulatory and the microscopic molecular genetic levels. Subsequent chapters will focus on the peripheral responses to the failing heart.

CONTRACTION AND RELAXATION OF THE HEART

Cardiac sarcomeres are the central elements of heart muscle contraction. Sarcomeres are joined end to end and aligned across the breadth of the cell, resulting in the characteristic striated appearance of the myocyte under the light microscope. The sarcomere contains two types of filaments that interdigitate and shorten during contraction: a thick filament made up of myosin and a thin filament made of actin. The thin filament also contains the proteins troponin and tropomyosin. All of these proteins are essential for contraction when appropriately activated. Actual shortening of the myocyte occurs as the thick and thin filaments couple and uncouple, producing a sliding motion across one another.

The cross-bridges are actually the heads of the myosin molecules protruding from the side of the thick filament. In the resting state, the actin sites, with which the myosin heads react, are blocked by tropomyosin; but during contraction, a sudden rise in intracellular calcium concentration triggers calcium–troponin C binding, which alters the configuration of the adjacent tropomyosin molecule. This exposes the specific myosin-binding site on the actin chain, allowing the myosin head to couple with the actin. Force is generated as the angle of this interaction changes, after which the couplet disengages; the process is repeated at a new, downstream actin site. Cardiac contraction can thus be described as a finely orchestrated rowing motion of the actin–myosin interaction, which depends on the calcium concentration.

Because calcium is essential for the cross-bridges to form and because the number of cross-bridges accounts for the power of contraction, contractility depends directly on the concentration of free calcium ions within the myocyte. The energy required for cross-bridge formation is supplied by adenosine triphosphate (ATP), which is broken down into inorganic phosphate (P_i) and adenosine diphosphate (ADP) by an enzyme localized in the myosin head. High concentrations of ATP are provided by the exceptionally high density of myocyte mitochondria, in which ATP is produced by oxidative phosphorylation. This is an obligatory oxygen-dependent process, which is why cardiac performance strongly depends on adequate coronary blood flow and the oxygen it supplies.

Unlike skeletal muscle, the heart is virtually incapable of anaerobic respiration. The release of calcium occurs from cisternal stores when electrical potentials cross the cell membrane. This is a complex and intricately regulated activity in and of itself. Undue attention is sometimes paid to the systolic activities of the myocyte and myocardium, but the heart must relax to fill and to set the stage for contraction. Diastole is also an energy-dependent activity, consuming approximately one-third of all energy stores used during the complete cardiac cycle. Of course, the heart must fill before it empties, and abnormalities of relaxation are just as important as those of contraction. The cycle of contraction and relaxation of the heart is an extraordinarily complicated symphony of intertwining harmonic themes that can be disrupted at myriad points to cause systolic and diastolic dysfunction, with subsequent heart failure.

MECHANISMS OF CARDIAC INJURY

Table 2.1 lists several mechanisms believed to be important when considering the cause of cardiac injury leading to heart failure and congestive states. Different diseases cause injury in different fashions, and individuals may be uniquely susceptible to the various disease processes. Heritable disorders produce molecular genetic

Table 2.1.   The Heart Failure Milieu: Routes of Myocardial Injury

Site	Mechanism	Examples
Nucleolar DNA	Heritable disorder	Muscular dystrophy; hypertrophic cardiomyopathy
Myocyte organelle	Perturbation in contractile protein production	Volume overload (MR, AI); pressure overload (HTN, AS)
Myocardial cell	Necrosis and apoptosis	Myocardial infarct; anthracycline toxicity; alcoholic cardiomyopathy

MR, mitral regurgitation; *AI*, aortic insufficiency; *HTN*, hypertension; *AS*, aortic stenosis.

alteration with subsequent contractile protein production abnormalities. For example, patients with muscular dystrophy–associated cardiomyopathy have myocardial injury originating from a heritable disorder. Patients with myotonic dystrophy and those with Duchenne muscular dystrophy frequently die of arrhythmias or heart failure caused by the cardiomyopathy rather than by skeletal muscle weakness. It has now been demonstrated that patients with hypertrophic cardiomyopathy have heritable disorders of troponin protein production, which lead to ventricular hypertrophy and inefficient systolic and diastolic cardiac function.

Volume or pressure overload produced by valvular insufficiency or stenosis, along with hypertension, induces abnormal molecular biodynamic activities, causing myocyte production to become more representative of the fetal than of the adult pattern (1–3). This results in myocyte contractile or relaxation abnormalities, which can ultimately impair systemic perfusion and cause metabolic disturbances that are characteristic of the heart failure syndrome. Diseases such as myocardial infarction, lymphocytic myocarditis, and anthracycline poisoning attack the myocyte itself causing premature cell death, sometimes acutely (e.g., anoxia from acute coronary thrombosis) and sometimes more slowly (e.g., the steady but accelerated myocyte demise by an up-regulated apoptosis program).

Table 2.2 lists specific diseases that the clinician might consider diagnosing when faced with a heart failure patient. The list adheres to the classification of cardiomyopathies suggested by the World

Health Organization and the International Society and Federation of Cardiology Task Force on the Definition and Classification of Cardiomyopathies (4). As suggested by the scheme, heart failure is grouped mainly into cardiomyopathies having certain anatomic characteristics (e.g., dilated, hypertrophic, and restrictive elements) or resulting from a specific injury (e.g., ischemic heart disease). It is important to consider the broad causal spectrum when evaluating patients, because many disease states that result in cardiomyopathy can be easily treated, with complete resolution of the heart failure syndrome (e.g., thyrotoxicosis and myxedema).

Dilated cardiomyopathy is characterized by marked multichamber cardiac enlargement, whereas hypertrophic cardiomyopathy patients have particularly small left ventricular cavity dimensions with marked muscular hypertrophy. Systolic function and contractility are usually markedly enhanced hypertrophic cardiomyopathy patients. Restrictive cardiomyopathy is characterized by more normal chamber size (at least with respect to the ventricles) but impaired relaxation or diastolic dysfunction that is not primarily the result of muscular hypertrophy in a classic sense. As Table 2.2 demonstrates, cardiomyopathies should be labeled by their causal factor as well as by their anatomic and physiologic correlates. Therefore, a patient with prior myocardial infarction, active ischemic heart disease, and substantive heart failure associated with congestion and a dilated left ventricle would correctly be labeled as having an ischemic dilated cardiomyopathy.

Obviously, multiple diseases can contribute to difficulties in a single patient. It is not particularly unusual to have a combination of ischemic heart disease and valvular heart disease (mitral regurgitation in a setting of prior inferolateral wall myocardial infarction, for example), or a combination of coronary heart disease, hypertension, and diabetes mellitus in a setting of significant congestive heart failure. It is challenging to determine which disease process is the primary one with respect to cause and exacerbation of the heart failure syndrome. One can never focus on a single disease entity in a vacuum, because myocardial injury can be caused by multiple comorbid conditions. When evaluating patients with heart failure, clinicians must first exclude treatable causes of the syndrome.

Today, when epidemiologic information and clinical trial participant data are reviewed, ischemic heart disease appears to account for the preponderance of patients with both asymptomatic left

Table 2.2.   Classification of Causes of Heart Failure

Dilated cardiomyopathy
- Idiopathic

Hypertrophic cardiomyopathy
- Idiopathic hypertrophic subaortic stenosis
- Hypertrophic obliterative cardiomyopathy
- Hypertrophic nonobstructive cardiomyopathy

Restrictive cardiomyopathy
- Specific infiltrating diseases
- Idiopathic

Arrhythmogenic right ventricular cardiomyopathy
- Idiopathic right ventricular outflow tract tachycardia
- Arrhythmogenic right ventricular dysplasia

Unclassifiable cardiomyopathies
- Atypical presentation
  - Fibroelastosis
  - Systolic dysfunction without dilation
  - Mitochondrial cardiomyopathy
- Mixed presentation (dilated, hypertrophic, restrictive)
- Amyloidosis (see *Metabolic*)
- Hypertension

Specific cardiomyopathies
- Ischemic
- Valvular obstruction or insufficiency
- Hypertensive
- Inflammatory
  - Myocarditis
  - Idiopathic lymphocytic
  - Giant cell
  - Autoimmune
  - Infectious
    - Chagas disease
    - Human immunodeficiency virus
    - Enterovirus
    - Adenovirus
    - Cytomegalovirus
    - Bacterial (endocarditis, myocarditis)

Metabolic
- Endocrine
  - Thyrotoxicosis
  - Hypothyroidism
  - Adrenal cortical insufficiency
  - Pheochromocytoma
  - Acromegaly
  - Diabetes mellitus
- Familial storage disease or infiltration
  - Hemochromatosis
  - Glycogen storage disease
  - Hurler syndrome
  - Refsum syndrome
- Niemann-Pick disease
  - Hand-Schüler-Christian disease
  - Fabry-Andersen disease
  - Morquio-Ullrich disease
- Deficiency
  - Potassium metabolism disturbances (hypokalemia)
  - Magnesium deficiency
- Nutritional disorders
  - Kwashiorkor
  - Anemia
  - Beriberi
  - Selenium deficiency
  - Nonspecific malabsorption or starvation
- Amyloid (primary, secondary, familial, hereditary, senile)
- Familial Mediterranean fever

General system disease
- Connective tissue disorders
  - Systemic lupus erythematosus
  - Polyarteritis nodose
  - Rheumatoid arthritis
  - Scleroderma
  - Dermatomyositis
  - Nonspecific infiltrations and granulomas
- Sarcoidosis
- Leukemia
- Muscular dystrophies
  - Duchenne
  - Becker
  - Myotonic

Table 2.2.   *(Continued)*

• Neuromuscular disorders • Friedreich ataxia • Noonan syndrome • Lentiginosis • Sensitivity and toxic reaction • Alcohol	• Catecholamines • Anthracyclines • Irradiation • Peripartal cardiomyopathy (a heterogeneous group)

Modified from World Health Organization/International Society and Federation of Cardiology Task Force on the Definition of Cardiomyopathies. 1995 report. *Circulation* 1996;93:8412–8420.

ventricular systolic dysfunction and congestive heart failure. Hypertension is frequently a comorbidity in these patients; and indeed, hypertension alone often takes second place to ischemic heart disease in these populations. Valvular heart disease, diabetic cardiomyopathy, and idiopathic dilated cardiomyopathy represent about a third of the heart failure population. Active myocarditis, or so-called viral cardiomyopathy, is actually rarely diagnosed with certainty. Whether patients with idiopathic cardiomyopathy had a preceding viral infection or inflammatory disease as the causal difficulty is a highly contentious subject and tenuous hypothesis. It is likely best for the clinician to focus on ischemic heart disease, hypertension, diabetes, and valvular heart disease as the primary causal factors of heart failure.

THE CARDIAC RESPONSE TO INJURY: NECROSIS, APOPTOSIS, AND HYPERTROPHY

Under normal conditions, cellular protein turnover is orderly and cardiac muscle–specific gene products replenish and repair contractile elements damaged during the normal wear and tear of cardiac contraction and relaxation (a cycle that occurs more than 100,000 times a day). Terminally differentiated postnatal cardiomyocytes do not seem capable of cell division; therefore, when the cell dies, it will not be replaced. It is important to remember that many of the contractile proteins and elements within the cell, however, regenerate every 30 to 90 days.

In the setting of a specific disease that leads to heart failure, myocyte membrane receptors are activated via increased load (mechanical stretch or pressure) and after humorally mediated receptor targets have been stimulated (5,6). This results in the shifting of protein synthesis to the fetal pattern, as noted above. It is likely that both the quantity of myocyte proteins, particularly of the contractile elements, and the quality of these peptides are adversely affected by the move toward fetal phenotypic expression (1). It is the increased production of myocellular organelle elements and proteins that leads to cellular hypertrophy and subsequent chamber dilation, the hallmarks of cardiac remodeling, which defines heart failure.

Table 2.3 summarizes some of the cell membrane receptors believed to be important in this process. Activation of these receptors in endocrine, paracrine, or autocrine fashion precipitates intracellular second messengers, such as cyclic adenosine monophosphate (cAMP) and inositol triphosphate, to induce a variety of intracellular enzyme mediators that then up regulate expression of excessive adult and fetal muscle cell–specific gene products. Unnatural growth of the cell follows, which results in myocardial hypertrophy and subsequent contractile and relaxing abnormalities. Large myocytes that express the fetal protein phenotype do not likely contract with normal vigor.

It has been speculated that apoptosis is triggered when a terminally differentiated cell, such as the adult myocyte, is excessively stimulated by the many growth hormones essential for myocyte regulatory homeostasis. The induction of hypertrophy, therefore,

Table 2.3.   Myocyte Cell Membrane Receptor Sites Likely Important in Heart Failure Remodeling

- Growth hormone
- Angiotensin II
- Norepinephrine, epinephrine
- Tumor necrosis factor
- Interleukin 1, 5, and 6
- Tissue-derived growth factors
- Endothelium-derived growth factors
- Platelet-derived growth factors
- Arginine vasopressin
- Nitric oxide
- Atrial natriuretic peptide

likely leads to cell loss via apoptosis, which, in turn, begins the self-perpetuating downward spiral of remodeling, clinical heart failure, humoral milieu perturbation, molecular biodynamic alteration, and further cell loss (7,8). Obviously, if acute injuries that lead to sudden cell necrosis are superimposed on this chronic, more insidious and subtle programmed cell death, the situation is worsened. Myocyte loss with the subsequent burden on the remaining contractile cells further perpetuates the cycle by leading to greater myocyte depletion and more cell death. There is an increasing pool of evidence suggesting that both cell necrosis and apoptosis are important in the life-and-death cycle of the cardiac myocyte.

As noted, *apoptosis* refers to cell death from the process of myocyte condensation, without disruption of the cell membrane, and the eventual fragmentation with pinocytosis of the cell contents and phagocytosis by neighboring cells. The term is well chosen. *Apoptosis* is a Greek word that characterizes the slow but steady falling away of petals from a flower's pistil. Table 2.4 summarizes the differences between myocyte necrosis, which is marked by cell surface membrane disruption, inflammation, and fibrotic replacement, and apoptosis. Although cell necrosis is commonly the result of myocardial infarction, viral or bacterial infection, and exposure to toxins (such adriamycin or alcohol), it is important to remember that triggering factors for apoptosis are less well characterized and are likely mediated by multiple mechanisms, including superoxide exposure, cytokines (e.g., tumor necrosis factor), and mechanical alteration of

Table 2.4.   Myocyte Necrosis Versus Apoptosis

Necrosis
- Cellular dropsy
- Mitochondrial swelling
- Loss of membrane integrity
- Random DNA degradation
- Inflammatory healing response

Apoptosis
- Cellular involution (shrinkage)
- No mitochondrial swelling
- Membrane initially remains intact
- Organized degradation of DNA (multiples of 180 base pair units)
- Little inflammatory response

myocyte geometry (as seen with excessive stretch or pressure). Obviously, we must continue to study these mechanisms so that therapies can be designed to block apoptotic activation sequences from either a receptor interdiction or a molecular genetic standpoint.

THE CARDIAC REMODELING PROCESS

Morphologically, myocardial hypertrophy is caused by an increased number of myofibrils and mitochondria and by the enlargement of mitochondria and the cell nucleus. An increase in intracellular disorganization ensues, which is ultimately characterized by the loss of contractile elements, disruption of Z-bands, interruption of the parallel arrangement of sarcomeres, and infiltration of fibrous tissue. Ventricular remodeling can then occur in two ways, depending on the type of stimulus, and are best characterized by the differences in remodeling induced by pressure compared to that induced by volume overload. Parallel sarcomere development and hypertrophy create concentric ventricular remodeling (whereby mass increases more than volume increases), whereas series sarcomere hypertrophy leads to eccentric remodeling (and volume increase is greater than mass increase). In both situations, compensatory hypertrophy develops in an attempt to maintain wall stress within normal calculated levels. Thus heart failure seen in a setting of hypertension (pressure overload) is characterized by small left ventricular chamber dimension, significant left ventricular muscle growth, and hypertrophy, with diastolic dysfunction or filling abnormalities predominating over reduced contractile performance. Eccentric hypertrophy is characteristic of long-standing and significant mitral insufficiency or aortic regurgitation, and ventricular dilation is the predominant observation. The massively enlarged heart, or cor bovinum, of chronic aortic insufficiency characterizes this nicely.

Detrimental effects of myocardial hypertrophy and dilation include increased wall stress, which is a major determinant of myocardial oxygen demand and alters the myocardial oxygen demand: supply ratio that characterizes cell energetics. Indeed, as noted, ventricular hypertrophy in and of itself contributes to myocardial blood flow disturbances (diminution). Finally, growth stimulators in terminally differentiated myocytes seem to be lethal to cells by triggering apoptosis.

Though it is important to focus on the myocyte, the cardiac interstitium should not be ignored (9). In response to the same mechanical, inflammatory, neurohumoral, and hormonal mediators of growth discussed above, cardiac interstitial matrix changes are also precipitated. The interstitium is composed primarily of collagen, elastin, glycoproteins, adrenergic nerve endings, blood and lymph vessels, mesenchymal cells (fibroblasts, pericytes, and macrophages) and fluid (an ultrafiltrate of plasma). Fibroblasts appear in the interstitium with greater frequency during wound healing and are seemingly essential to fibrogenesis and remodeling of the noncellular matrix. Inflammatory cells are also important in this process, increasing in concentration and intensity after myocyte injury.

One great challenge is to differentiate between interstitial inflammatory processes that are a normal part of cardiac repair and maintenance from processes likely to be associated with pathologic conditions. By its very nature, the myocardial interstitial matrix is resistant to stretch during diastole and, therefore, contributes to limitations in ventricular dilation and, in large part, is responsible for the pathologic stiffness associated with diastolic dysfunction. It has been suggested that there is a reciprocal regulation of collagen turnover in cardiovascular tissues with stimulators of fibrosis, including angiotensin II, transforming growth factor β, and endothelin 1 and 3. Inhibitors of fibrosis include bradykinin, prostaglandins, and nitric oxide. When stimulated, the interstitial matrix laydown system increases collagen synthesis, reduces collagenase activity, and stiffens the entire support matrix, possibly to a pathophysiologic degree.

MYOCYTE MEMBRANE RECEPTOR RESPONSES

Because the therapeutic paradigm in heart failure is shifting toward the use of β-adrenergic blockers in many patients, it is important to specifically consider the myocyte membrane responses noted in these patients. As part of the cardiac response to injury, membrane receptors may be significantly altered in concentration and function (10–14). Like other cellular elements, internal and external membrane receptors are regulated in terms of density and function by the molecular biodynamics of the cell. Adrenergic receptors include both α- and β-adrenergic families; and each receptor pathway elicits a variety of biochemical and physiologic activities, which are either antagonistic or additive to the activity of other receptors. Furthermore, the cardiac effects of α- and β-adrenergic receptors must be viewed in conjunction with their effects on peripheral circulation (discussed in Chapter 3).

Although there are several categories of α-adrenergic receptors, only α_1-receptors demonstrate significant myocardial density. These receptors modulate change in intracellular cytoplasmic calcium concentration and control or affect several important parameters. Stimulation of α_1-adrenergic receptor pathways modulates heart rate, myocardial contractility; wall tension; and systolic, diastolic, and peripheral vascular compliance. The density of α_1-receptors increases modestly in settings of heart failure, and it has been hypothesized that this eventually results in greater myocardial hypertrophy. Stimulation of α_1-receptors also likely increases cardiac dysrhythmia.

β-adrenergic receptors are linked to intracellular G protein–signaling pathways and are important in modulating adenyl cyclase activity, which, ultimately, is critical to inotropic, chronotropic, and lusitropic activities. It appears that in the heart failure setting, selective down regulation of β_1-adrenergic receptors is noted, without much detectable change in β_2-receptor activity. This down regulation of β_1-adrenergic receptors alters the β_1- and β_2-subtype populations, which may affect the choice of β-adrenergic receptor blocking agent prescribed to patients with heart failure. This issue is reviewed in Chapter 4, in which data from clinical trials evaluating various therapeutic strategies are summarized.

SUMMARY

Heart failure results from myocyte injury, and compensatory processes evolve in an initial attempt to maintain cellular homeostasis. It is the initial loading change foisted on normal or relatively normal myocytes that leads to the molecular responses that ultimately account for ventricular remodeling. Ventricular remodeling is most generally and, perhaps, best characterized as myocardial hypertrophy, with cardiac chamber dilation and increased interstitial matrix formation. Physiologically, remodeling is an attempt to maintain low wall stress while ensuring that contractile power imparts adequate circulatory flow to peripheral organs and tissues.

Indeed, compensation marks the second stage of heart failure, during which stroke volume is reasonable enough to maintain adequate systemic perfusion, although a variety of humors are released. Subsequent molecular genetic and circulatory system perturbations are noted. Cardiac remodeling continues toward the final stages of heart failure characterized by progressive left ventricular dysfunction, further hypertrophy, fibrotic infiltration of cardiac muscle and interstitium, and cell necrosis or induction of an apoptosis program.

It is important to recognize that the earliest stages of heart failure can be present in asymptomatic patients who have only subtle molecular biodynamic changes, which are secondary to the difficult-to-detect myocyte load alteration. Manifest heart failure develops only late in the progression of the syndrome, when it is characterized by an even greater degree of ventricular remodeling and more obvious peripheral circulatory and physiologic abnormalities.

REFERENCES

1. Parker TG, Schneider MD. Growth factors, proto-oncogenes, and plasticity of the cardiac phenotype. Annu Rev Physiol 1991;53:179–200.
2. Pollack P. Proto-oncogenes and the cardiovascular system. Chest 1995;107:826–835.
3. Feldman AM, Ray PE, Silan CM, et al. Selective gene expression in failing human heart: quantification of steady-state levels of messenger RNA in endomyocardial biopsies using the polymerase chain reaction. Circulation 1991;83:1866–1872.
4. World Health Organization/International Society and Federation Task Force on the Definition of Cardiomyopathies. 1995 report. Circulation 1996;93:8412–8420.
5. Sadoshima J, Xu Y, Slayter HS, Izumo S. Autocrine release of angiotensin II mediates stretch-induced hypertrophy of cardiac myocytes in vitro. Cell 1993;75:977–984.
6. Rozich JD, Barnes MA, Schmid PG, et al. Load effect on gene expression during cardiac hypertrophy. J Mol Cell Cardiol 1995;27:485–499.
7. Narula J, Haider N, Virmani R, et al. Apoptosis in myocytes in end-stage heart failure. N Engl J Med 1996;335:1182–1189.
8. Yeh ETH. Life and death in the cardiovascular system. Circulation 1997;95:782–786.
9. Weber KT. Cardiac interstitium. In: Wilson-Poole PA, Colucci WS, Massie BM, et al., eds., Heart failure: scientific principles and clinical practice. New York: Churchill Livingstone, 1997.
10. Bristow MR, Anderson FL, Port JD, et al. Differences in β-adrenergic neuroeffector mechanisms in ischemic vs. idiopathic dilated cardiomyopathy. Circulation 1991;84:1024–1039.
11. Studer R, Reinecke H, Bilger J, et al. Gene expression of the cardiac Na^+–Ca^{2+} exchanger in end-stage human heart failure. Circ Res 1994;75:443–453.

12. Bristow MR, Ginsburg R, Minobe W, et al. Decreased catecholamine sensitivity and beta-adrenergic receptor density in failing human hearts. N Engl J Med 1982;307:205–211.
13. Fowler MB, Laser JA, Hopkins GL, et al. Assessment of the beta-adrenergic receptor pathway in the intact failing human heart: progressive receptor down-regulation and subsensitivity to agonist response. Circulation 1986;74:1290–1302.
14. Bristow MR. Changes in myocardial and vascular receptors in heart failure. J Am Coll Cardiol 1993;61A–71A.

Chapter 3

Circulatory and Physiologic Responses in Heart Failure

James B. Young

CIRCULATORY RESPONSE TO HEART FAILURE

The result of myocardial injury, with its compensatory remodeling, is an alteration in ventricular function and the subsequent impaired contraction and relaxation. Changes can range from subtle perturbation to dramatic and clinically overt performance abnormalities (1–3). A wide range of mitigating circumstances influences the presentation of symptoms in patients with heart failure. Depending on the principal location of injury, predominance of diastolic or systolic dysfunction, circulatory system integrity, aerobic cardiovascular conditioning, and treatments used, various hemodynamic, neurohormonal, humoral, and inflammatory reactions occur. It is, however, reduced stroke volume—an essential element of the syndrome—that triggers the peripheral flow derangements that are largely responsible for altering normal neurohormonal and humoral circulatory homeostasis.

A complicated positive and negative feedback loop interaction occurs among peripheral receptors in the vascular network, the central nervous system, and the solid organs, such as the kidney (4–7). The autonomic nervous system is largely responsible for much of this flow control (4). Autonomic balance is coordinated by the afferent nervous system, which signals from peripheral baroreceptors located in the heart, lungs, and great vessels. Chemoreceptors, located in the carotid bodies and skeletal muscle, and sensory receptors, located in the skin and other visceral organs, monitor oxygen saturation, carbon dioxide levels, and acid–base balance and thus contribute to afferent signaling as well. When flows are altered, tissue perfusion homeostasis is maintained by a variety of vasodilating and vasoconstricting responses.

From a teleologic viewpoint, these systems evolved, in large part, to maintain circulatory compensation in settings of significant dehydration or hemorrhagic volume loss. The life expectancy of prehistoric humans was short, and mortality was largely related to the ability to compensate for traumatic injury, diseases causing hypovolemia, and extremes of nutritional deprivation. It seems that longer-living modern humans have acquired different diseases much more quickly than these compensatory systems have evolved to more appropriately compensate. That which is likely advantageous and beneficial for the immediate maintenance of circulatory homeostasis after traumatic blood loss can be detrimental over the long term in heart failure patients. Indeed, the pathophysiologic process of heart failure is associated with the dysfunction of the baroreceptors and chemoreceptors, accounting for the increased sympathetic and reduced parasympathetic nervous system activity seen in this setting.

It is the baroreceptor activity that principally modulates nervous system tone during changes in intravascular volume or pressure. Cardiopulmonary baroreceptors in the heart and pulmonary vasculature, the aortic arch, and the carotid sinus (arterial baroreceptors) produce afferent neurosignals to the central nervous system via the vagus and glossopharyngeal nerves. Normally, these signals inhibit sympathetic and augment parasympathetic nervous system efferent activity. In situations of volume depletion or hypotension, decreased receptor stimulation by reduced arterial wall stretch diminishes the afferent signaling, thereby decreasing parasympathetic activity and increasing sympathetic stimulation, which is then associated with increased epinephrine and norepinephrine release. As a result of the baroreceptor dysfunction noted in heart failure patients, efferent inhibitory input is decreased, leading to excessive sympathetic and diminished parasympathetic nervous system activity. Clinically, this is manifest by increased venous and arterial tone, higher systemic vascular resistance, increased heart rate, and decreased electrocardiographic RR interval variability, which is a surrogate marker of parasympathetic tone. All of these observations have been related to the insidious progression of heart failure and associated with an adverse outcome.

It is also likely that baroreceptor function facilitates vasopressin release from the midbrain neurohypothesis, with its subsequent stimulation of renal renin release. Circulating renin is primarily released from the juxtaglomerular apparatus of the kidney. Many factors combine to trigger this systemic release, including increased renal sympathetic nervous system efferent activity, decreased distal tubular sodium delivery, reduced renal perfusion pressure, and diuretic therapy. Atrial natriuretic factor (ANF) may inhibit the release of renin.

Renin is responsible for cleaving angiotensinogen, a tetrapeptide produced in the liver, to the inactive peptide angiotensin I (AI). AI is subsequently converted to AII by angiotensin-converting enzyme (ACE); this reaction occurs principally in the lung. In addition to the systemic conversion pathway, other systems are likely present in tissues (such as the heart), where proteases (such as chymase) seem to be responsible for producing AII via an ACE-independent pathway. AII is a powerful vasoconstrictor and promotes sodium reabsorption by inducing aldosterone secretion by directly affecting tubular reabsorption of salt. AII also stimulates water intake by increasing thirst and facilitates the release of norepinephrine by stimulating sympathetic nerve endings.

Many studies have now demonstrated that plasma norepinephrine, epinephrine, renin, vasopressin, and atrial natriuretic peptide levels are increased in a graded fashion when heart failure is noted. The worse the clinical heart failure syndrome, generally, the higher the level of these hormones. It is important to stress that disturbance of the neurohumoral milieu can be demonstrated in patients with asymptomatic left ventricular systolic dysfunction and in those with manifest congestive heart failure.

At the core of circulatory regulation is the sympathetic nerve terminal, with neurotransmitter release at the sympathetic neuroeffector junction being modulated by a variety of hormones and other substances that act on the receptors located at the presynaptic nerve ending. Several endogenous and exogenous α_2-adrenergic receptor agonists (such as opioids, prostanoids, purines, histamines, 5-hydroxytryptamine, ANF, dopamine, and acetylcholine) inhibit norepinephrine release, whereas epinephrine and AII increase norepinephrine release from the neuroeffector junction. Although peripheral blood flow is largely determined by interactions among sympathetic efferent nerve signals, several autoregulatory systems are also active and important in the peripheral circulation. Endothelium-derived relaxing factor (EDRF), endothelin, prostaglandin, kinins and mechanical factors (such as muscle activity and cutaneous thermoregulation) can affect systemic blood flow.

Vasoconstricting systems thus include the sympathetic nervous system, the renin–angiotensin–aldosterone system, arginine vasopressin, and endothelin; and counterposing vasodilating systems are stimulated by ANF, the kallikrein–kinin system, vasodilating prostaglandin, and EDRF. These feedback loops are stimulated or inhibited by varying degrees of vasoconstriction or vasodilation, which are sensed locally (Table 3.1).

Recently, proinflammatory cytokines—interleukin 1 (IL-1), IL-6, and tumor necrosis factor α (TNF-α)—have been discovered to play a significant role in patients with heart failure, and particularly in those with more advanced syndromes (8). As congestive heart failure worsens, high systemic levels of TNF-α are seen, and a relationship exists between other perturbed neurohormonal systems and the level of proinflammatory cytokines detected. Higher levels of TNF-α have been associated with diminished survival in some clinical trials (9). Furthermore, TNF-α has been demonstrated to be a potent negative inotropic humor, and it is now known that this cytokine is

Table 3.1.   Humoral Factors in Heart Failure Important in Regulation of Vascular Circulation

Vasoconstricting factors[a]
- Renin–angiotensin–aldosterone
- Epinephrine–norepinephrine
- Neuropeptide Y
- Vasopressin
- Endothelin
- Thromboxane

Vasodilating factors[b]
- Prostaglandin
- Natriuretic peptides
- Kinens
- Nitric oxide (endothelial-derived relaxing factor)
- Vasoactive intestinal peptide
- Calcitonin-related peptide
- Substance P
- Endorphins

[a] Primary antinatriuretic and may stimulate or accelerate myocyte growth or hypertrophy.
[b] Largely natriuretic and may inhibit or reverse myocyte growth or hypertrophy.

actually produced by the myocardium as a response to increased afterload.

Though initially believed important only in cardiac cachexia, it appears that cytokines play a much broader role in the pathophysiologic process and perpetuation of the heart failure syndrome. Obviously, many targets can be identified that are based on perturbation of these neurohormonal, humeral, and inflammatory systems active in heart failure patients (2). ACE inhibitors, AII receptor blockers, α-adrenergic blockers, β-adrenergic blockers, and endothelin antagonists are examples of drugs used either routinely or experimentally in heart failure patients today. Therapies of this sort, obviously, have not been designed primarily to augment contractility or induce diuresis in the heart failure patient but rather to interdict more fundamental system abnormalities.

SYSTEMIC ORGAN RESPONSES TO HEART FAILURE

Pulmonary Congestion

Because of the intimate interrelationship between cardiac and pulmonary function with respect to anatomy and physiologic processes, it is not surprising that pulmonary abnormalities quickly appear in heart failure patients whose symptoms include congestion (10). Reduction in peak expiratory flow rate (PEFR), forced expiratory volume (FEV), and the expiratory volume:vital capacity ratio are all well described in settings of congestive heart failure. Acute bronchospasm, or cardiac asthma, is a frightening complication of acute pulmonary edema; it generally can be quickly resolved with aggressive diuresis and vasodilator therapy designed to lower pulmonary pressures and, specifically, pulmonary capillary wedge pressure (PCWP). Even in the absence of significant pulmonary edema, however, reduction in FEV and vital capacity (VC) are noted and are related to symptomatic severity. These restrictive pulmonary defects correlate directly with peak exercise oxygen uptake (11). Chronic changes in bronchovascular sheath anatomy secondary to chronic pulmonary venous hypertension and submucosal edema likely cause the reduced airway caliber noted in congestive heart failure patients, which leads to the restrictive and obstructive pulmonary abnormalities. Reduction in the pulmonary diffusing capacity for carbon monoxide has also been shown, and this contributes to gas exchange abnormalities in the setting of heart failure. Pulmonary gas diffusion limitation appears to be caused by reduction in lung volume secondary to cardiomegaly and intrathoracic venous volume and by inherent membrane diffusion abnormalities, which have not been completely characterized.

The mechanical and diffusion abnormalities characteristic of heart failure are responsible, in large part, for exertional dyspnea. Indeed, increased ventilatory response is one of the hallmarks of congestive heart failure; ventilatory levels are higher than expected at any given workload or level of carbon dioxide production. Abnormalities in intrinsic pulmonary gas exchange are further exacerbated by deficiencies observed in respiratory skeletal muscle function. Respiratory muscle strength is reduced in patients with severely symptomatic congestive heart failure and correlates with their complaints of dyspnea and with peak exercise oxygen uptake. Furthermore, deoxygenation of respiratory muscles occurs during exercise even when significant arterial deoxygenation is absent. This contributes to the dyspnea and fatigue of chronic congestive heart failure. Reasons for this uncoupling of muscle performance and the circulatory system are not well understood. Also contributing to the ventilation abnormalities noted in this population is increased dead space ventilation.

Thus many interrelated difficulties—increased pulmonary artery and venous pressures, pulmonary vasculature edema, airway luminal narrowing, diminished lung volume, impaired gas transfer, and respiratory muscle inadequacy—contribute to the symptoms in heart failure. Further complicating these issues are pulmonary comorbid conditions, such as chronic obstructive pulmonary disease, interstitial fibrosis, and pulmonary infection.

Exercise Capacity

Exercise intolerance is noted as the chronic heart failure syndrome worsens, and it is particularly problematic in patients with congestive heart failure (11). Symptoms of dyspnea and muscle fatigue, resulting in generalized weakness, are initially seen only during extreme exertion. As the syndrome progresses, less stress is needed to precipitate symptoms; and in the worst stages of heart failure, the symptoms are present even at rest. Exercise intolerance is influenced by abnormalities at several levels, including the lungs, skeletal muscle, peripheral resistance vessels, and vascular endothelium. Indeed, abnormalities of mitochondrial function in skeletal muscles have been observed in congestive heart failure patients. Although indices such as left ventricular ejection fraction, left ventricular dimension, and hemodynamics frequently correlate with prognosis in heart failure, they do not necessarily relate precisely to exercise tolerance and maximal oxygen uptake.

Obviously, exercise places additional demands on the heart and circulatory system, because of the increase in oxygen-dependent metabolic energy requirements and in cellular respiratory waste products that need to be eliminated. During exercise, cardiac output demands are 5–10 times greater than those needed at rest. Theoretically, normal subjects have a well-integrated oxygen delivery pathway, which moves oxygen from the ambient air to the skeletal muscle mitochondria and quickly and efficiently carries carbon dioxide and acid byproducts of respiration to the expired air or urine.

Healthy subjects rarely have a limitation in exercise capacity that is precipitated by pulmonary function limitations. The most common limitation to exercise is the inability of the heart to pump an adequate amount of blood peripherally; however, skeletal muscle energy substrate use is now known to be important and a significant rate-limiting factor as well. These peripheral systems are perturbed in patients with heart failure; therefore, it is not solely a limitation in the maximal cardiac output capacity that causes exercise intolerance in these patients.

To reiterate, factors in the heart failure patient that contribute to exercise limitation include perturbation of respiratory muscle function, diminished oxygen-diffusing capacity of the alveolar membrane, peripheral vascular changes that impair delivery of oxygenated blood to the muscles, attenuated oxygen extraction by the skeletal muscles, reduction in the oxidative capacity of muscle mitochondria, altered extraction of lactate and carbon dioxide, and the ability of the patient to tolerate dyspnea. We know that in many normal subjects, these physiologic functions can be improved with aerobic conditioning. Indeed, preconditioning appears to protect individuals when heart failure occurs.

One method of quantifying the severity of heart failure is to determine the patient's exercise capacity. Although there is a correlation between oxygen consumption and work levels in patients with heart failure, the relationship is not direct enough to reliably estimate oxygen consumption, particularly after anaerobic metabolism develops, via extrapolations from workload achieved during simple exercise testing. When efforts are made to determine objectively oxygen consumption and carbon dioxide production during graded workload stress, information is more reproducible and reliable. Maximum oxygen consumption ($\dot{V}o_2$max) during exercise relates to the functional activity classification, as assessed by New York Heart Association (NYHA) criteria, which correlates with patient prognosis and beneficial responses to therapy. Whether $\dot{V}o_2$max should be routinely used in heart failure patients has yet to be clarified. Cardiopulmonary exercise testing clearly plays an important role in selecting patients for more radical treatment, such as cardiac transplantation and ventricular assist device implantation; and it has been particularly important in giving us great insight into the pathophysiologic process of heart failure.

The Congestive State

As has been emphasized, heart failure is a broad category that includes patients without significant symptoms to those who are dyspneic and fatigued at rest, with profound dropsy or cardiogenic shock and circulatory collapse. Historically, a great deal of attention has been focused on the congestive state resulting from heart failure. Most patients with heart failure, however, do not spend most of their days significantly volume overloaded. Because volume overload does occur and contributes to the pulmonary, vascular, and skeletal muscle aberrations noted in more advanced heart failure, this component of the milieu must be put into perspective.

The kidneys' response to circulatory, neurologic, humoral, and hormonal changes triggered by heart failure contributes to the volume overload noted in congestive heart failure patients (7). Indeed, the kidneys are exquisitely sensitive to circulatory volume and solute composition and are normally able to regulate these parameters within tight limits. Both extrarenal and intrarenal mechanisms affect the kidneys' ability to maintain body fluid composition and volume. Factors important in renal solute and water handling can be classified as belonging to either afferent sensor or afferent effector volume regulatory systems. At the core of this activity is a change in tubular sodium and water absorption or excretion, which results in salt and water retention states. Vasoconstrictor neurohormonal activation signals the kidney to retain salt and water, which appears to be mediated by cardiac and vascular baroceptor stimulation of the sympathetic nervous system, which leads to activation of the renin–angiotensin–aldosterone system and the release of vasopressin as a response to diminishing organ perfusion and blood pressure. Countermanding vasodilator actions of prostaglandins and various natriuretic peptides are responsible for ameliorating some of the adverse effects of vasoconstriction.

The administration of diuretics, vasodilators, and neurohumoral blocking agents will, of course, affect the degree of salt and water retention occurring at any given time in any specific patient. Table 3.2 summarizes the renal effects of neurohormonal activation in heart failure and relates these actions to physiologic responses that, ultimately, result in hypervolemia; hyponatremia; and disordered magnesium, potassium, and chloride handling.

Table 3.2.   Renal Effects of Neurohormonal Activation in Heart Failure Patients

Vasoconstrictor Activities
- Renin–angiotensin–aldosterone
  - Angiotensin II
    - Efferent greater than afferent arteriolar constriction
    - Enhances sodium reabsorption in proximal tubule
    - Stimulates adrenal aldosterone synthesis and release
  - Aldosterone
    - Enhances sodium reabsorption with potassium secretion in collecting duct
  - Arginine vasopressin
    - Increases water reabsorption in medullary collecting duct
    - Increases sodium chloride reabsorption in medullary ascending limb of Henle's loop

Vasodilator Activities
- Atrial natriuretic peptide
  - Increases glomerular filtration rate
  - Promotes diminished sodium reabsorption in collecting duct
  - Suppresses renin activity
  - Inhibits aldosterone synthesis and release
  - Inhibits vasopressin release
- Renal prostaglandins
  - Promote renal vasodilation
  - Decrease tubular sodium reabsorption in ascending limb of Henle's loop
  - Inhibit vasopressin action in collecting duct

SUMMARY

The physiologic responses to the altered contraction and relaxation cycle of cardiac pump function depend on multiple and diverse feedback loop systems that are redundant and intimately interrelated. Although the initial response is an attempt to maintain circulatory homeostasis and adequate oxygenated blood supply to vital organs, the chronic perpetuation of neurohumoral, hormonal, and inflammatory responses sets the stage for continued cardiac injury and dysfunction. The systemic failure of the cardiovascular system to maintain adequate nutrient delivery to sustain peripheral cellular respiration activities and remove waste products leads to the congestive state of chronic heart failure, which contributes to the dyspnea syndromes and activity intolerance noted in late stages.

REFERENCES

1. Young JB, Pratt CM. Hemodynamic and hormonal alterations in patients with heart failure: toward a contemporary definition of heart failure. Semin Nephrol 1994;14:427–440.
2. Young JB. Overview of medical therapy in heart failure: the challenge of rational polypharmacy. In: Balady GJ, Pina IL, eds., Exercise and heart failure. Mt. Kisco, NY: Futura, 1997.
3. Young JB, Farmer JA. The diagnostic evaluation of patients with heart failure. In: Hosenpud JD, Greenberg BH, eds., Congestive heart failure; pathophysiology, diagnosis, and comprehensive approach to management. New York: Springer-Verlag, 1994:597–621.
4. Colucci WS. The sympathetic nervous system in congestive heart failure. In: Hosenpud JD, Greenberg BH, eds., Congestive heart failure; pathophysiology, diagnosis, and comprehensive approach to management. New York: Springer-Verlag, 1994:126–135.
5. Packer M. Nonadrenergic hormonal alterations in congestive heart failure. In: Hosenpud JD, Greenberg BH, eds., Congestive heart failure; pathophysiology, diagnosis, and comprehensive approach to management. New York: Springer-Verlag, 1994:136–144.
6. Hirsch AT, Creager MA. The peripheral circulation in heart failure. In: Hosenpud JD, Greenberg BH, eds., Congestive heart failure; pathophysiology, diagnosis, and comprehensive approach to management. New York: Springer-Verlag, 1994:145–160.
7. Abraham WT, Schrier RW. Renal salt and water handling in congestive heart failure. In: Hosenpud JD, Greenberg BH, eds., Congestive heart failure; pathophysiology, diagnosis, and comprehensive approach to management. New York: Springer-Verlag, 1994:161–177.
8. Mann DL, Young JB. Basic mechanisms in congestive heart failure: recognizing the role of proinflammatory cytokines. Chest 1994;105:897–904.
9. Torre-Amione G, Kapadia S, Lee J, et al. Pro-inflammatory cytokine levels in patients with depressed left ventricular ejection fraction: a report from the studies of left ventricular dysfunction (SOLVD). J Am Coll Cardiol 1996;27:1201–1206.
10. Puri P, Cleland JGF. The effects of chronic heart failure on pulmonary function. In: McMurray JJV, Cleland JGF, eds., Heart failure in clinical practice. St. Louis: Mosby, 1996:123–134.
11. Chua TP, Coats AJS. Which exercise test, if any? In: McMurray JJV, Cleland JGF, eds., Heart failure in clinical practice. St. Louis: Mosby, 1996:171–188.

Chapter 4

Altered Loading in Heart Failure

Andrew M. Cross Jr. and Roger M. Mills Jr.

Congestive heart failure as a result of left ventricular systolic dysfunction reflects myocardial injury, leading to a depressed contractile state. In response to depressed cardiac performance and decreased cardiac output, the body takes steps to maintain normal perfusion to vital organs (e.g., the brain). Decreased cardiac output reflexly activates the sympathetic nervous system and the renin—angiotensin–aldosterone endocrine volume-regulatory response, the neurohumoral aspect of heart failure. This response is linked to hemodynamic changes: renal sodium and water retention increases preload, sympathetic α-adrenergic vasoconstriction increases afterload, and myocardial inotropic β-adrenergic stimulation increases the contractile state and drives tachycardia. In the short term, a normal forward cardiac output is maintained. In the long term, the increased loads on an already dysfunctional heart lead to further deterioration of cardiac performance. A progressive spiral of increased loading, worsening fluid retention, and overt cardiac failure results in the syndrome of symptomatic congestive heart failure.

Any discussion of the hemodynamics of heart failure must deal with the critical issues of systolic and diastolic cardiac parameters and the relationship of volume versus pressure work performed. Understanding the modern therapy of heart failure demands a commitment from the physician to deal with these issues in enough detail to have a sense of why, at the mechanical level, certain interventions work to help patients feel better and why others do not. This chapter first reviews the physiologic determinants of heart function as understood via the classic ventricular function curve. The concept of mitral regurgitation in heart failure is then explored, to set hemodynamic

41

goals for therapy. Finally, the therapeutic role of positive inotropic agents is revisited as related to the defined treatment end points.

DETERMINANTS OF CARDIAC PERFORMANCE

The four major determinants of cardiac performance reflected by stroke volume are preload, afterload, heart rate, and contractile state. Braunwald et al. (1) outlined the definitions of *preload* and *afterload* in an early textbook, which lead to the widespread acceptance and eventual clinical use of the terms as synonyms for venous filling pressure and systolic pressure.

Ventricular preload, defined in the intact heart as wall stress or tension present at end-diastole, is reflected for clinical purposes by the left ventricular end-diastolic pressure (LVEDP). Pulmonary capillary wedge pressure (PCWP), obtained by right heart catheterization, mimics the LVEDP in the absence of significant pulmonary vascular disease or obstruction to left ventricular (LV) inflow. The ventricular filling pressures depend on the volume of venous return and ventricular compliance. Ventricular afterload, in strictest terms, encompasses the wall stress or tension generated during systole and is, therefore, shape dependent. Clinically, however, *afterload* connotes the resistance to antegrade ejection of volume into the systemic circulation—systemic vascular resistance (SVR)—which can be defined by the highly simplified resistance equation:

$$SVR = Arterial\ blood\ pressure/Cardiac\ output$$

The Ventricular Function Curve

Ventricular function curves relate systolic to diastolic performance. The term *Starling curve* or *Frank-Starling curve* is often applied to the graph of ventricular filling pressure versus cardiac output, which most physicians recognize as the typical ventricular function curve. In heart failure, the normal curve, shown in Figure 4.1, is shifted downward and to the right and is flattened. The effects of intervention are also shown in the figure. Volume reduction with diuretics or other measures can reduce filling pressures but have little effect on systolic performance, because of the flat shape of the curve. Positive inotropic agents, or afterload reduction, help restore the curve to a more normal configuration.

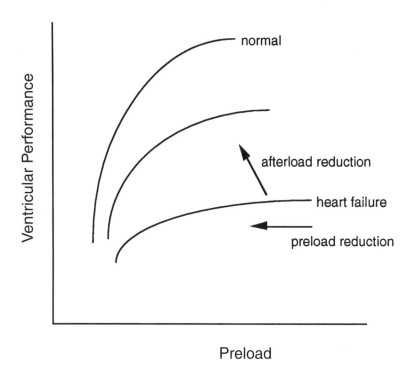

Figure 4.1:   Typical ventricular function curve. Modified from Braunwald E, Ross J Jr, Sonnenblick EH. Mechanisms of contraction of the normal and failing heart, 2nd ed. Boston: Little, Brown, 1976.

As can be seen on the ventricular function curve, in the absence of changes in afterload, increases in preload can increase cardiac output. Because the vascular circulation is a closed system, however, changes in one component of load will affect the other component, indicating that preload and afterload are coupled. Thus altering systemic blood pressure can influence overall cardiac performance (by causing a shift in the ventricular function curve) and induce a change in ventricular filling pressures. The contractile state and heart rate influence cardiac output, independent of loading conditions.

Although this scheme was developed from observations of papillary muscle strips that were treated with cardiodepressant compounds in the laboratory, it may apply to at least some forms of clinical acute heart failure. However, as illustrated in Figure 4.2,

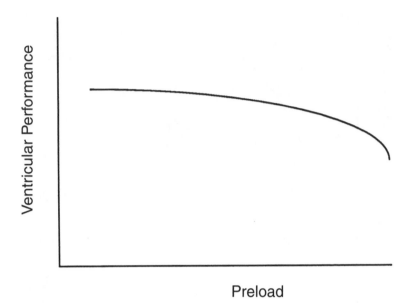

Figure 4.2: Response of a patient with chronic heart failure to diuretic and vasodilator therapy differs qualitatively from responses seen in patients with acute heart failure. Modified from Stevenson LW, Tillisch JH. Maintenance of cardiac output with normal filling pressures in patients with dilated heart failure. Circulation 1986:74:1303–1308.

Stevenson et al. (3,4) have shown that the response of the chronic heart failure patient to diuretic and vasodilator therapy differs qualitatively from the findings in the acute setting. In the chronic setting, effective reduction of the resistance against which the failing ventricle ejects leads to incremental improvement in forward flow far beyond what one might expect from muscle mechanics alone. The improvement is associated with an absolute decrease in filling pressure, which, from classical muscle mechanics analysis, should decrease performance. How is this physiologic legerdemain accomplished?

Redistribution of Mitral Regurgitant Flow with Afterload Reduction

Chronic left ventricular chamber dilation is often associated with significant mitral regurgitation (MR), which adversely contributes to the decline in overall cardiac performance. Several lines of evidence converge to suggest that the primary mechanism involved in the simultaneous enhancement of forward flow and drop in filling pressures seen with vasodilator therapy represents a redistribution of mitral regurgitant flow. These studies include the hemodynamic evidence outlined above; Konstam et al.'s (5) radionuclide scintigraphic studies, which show reduction of regurgitant flow with vasodilators; and our echocardiographic studies from pretransplant patients, which infer that severe functional MR on maximal therapy is a good predictor of a poor long-term prognosis.

Clinically, the neurohormonal response to worsening heart failure includes at least three different physiologic effects, which converge to initiate and then foster worsening functional MR: *(a)* expansion of extracellular volume in response to hypoperfusion, *(b)* increased peripheral vascular resistance, and *(c)* tachycardia.

Expansion of circulating volume distends the diseased LV, further stretching the mitral annulus and the mitral apparatus, altering the internal geometry of the papillary muscles, and ultimately redirecting the vector forces of their contraction to foster central regurgitation rather than buttress the valve leaflets against the force of LV systolic pressure. In addition, as volume expansion occurs, LV diastolic pressure rises and the pressure gradient available for diastolic perfusion of the subendocardium becomes compromised.

At the same time, peripheral resistance rises, thus changing the relative resistances that determine the distribution of total LV stroke volume between the open aortic valve and the functionally regurgitant mitral valve. With redistribution of systolic flow into the left atrium, atrial pressure rises and forward output falls, perpetuating the pathophysiologic cycle.

Finally, with increasing sympathetic tone in response to poor perfusion, the heart rate rises. Tachycardia, as a primary determinant of myocardial oxygen need, then taxes the coronary circulation to deliver more metabolic substrate to the functioning myocardium; simultaneously, the rising diastolic pressures, as noted above, diminish the perfusion gradient available to generate effective coronary flow.

This self-perpetuating cycle of worsening functional mitral regurgitation and advancing heart failure helps explain conceptually the natural history of the disease that we see clinically. Early mild heart failure progresses slowly for 2 or 3 years, responsive to modest doses of diuretics; but inevitably, patients who survive deteriorate into a cycle of relentlessly worsening failure in which the options narrow to intractable edema or prerenal azotemia and chronic severe volume depletion.

HEMODYNAMIC OBJECTIVES OF THERAPY

With this overview of the chronic heart failure patient's physiologic dilemma, the objectives of afterload reduction therapy become clear. The hemodynamic goals of therapy should include the following. (a) Reduction of peripheral vascular resistance to the lowest levels consistent with adequate perfusion of brain and kidneys to maximize forward output and minimize chronic mitral regurgitation. (b) Reduction of volume overload to achieve an edema-free state at levels of pulmonary pressure that maintain sufficient preload to maintain cardiac output. (c) Stabilization of heart rate in a range that allows adequate volume flow over time without resting tachycardia and with an appropriate rate response to modest activity.

Altering the adverse loading conditions allows the heart to better compensate for its decreased contractility and may also promote some degree of recovery by allowing the heart to rest. When contractility is depressed, the shape of the ventricular function curve is flattened and shifted to the right. In this circumstance, preload reduction can markedly decrease wall stress, resulting in decreased afterload and improved performance by actually shifting the curve upward and to the left. Congestion resolves with improved cardiac output. Diuretics are effective in reducing preload and congestion by decreasing intravascular volume. In addition, nitrates are peripheral venodilators and reduce preload by decreasing venous return.

Arterial vasodilators reduce afterload by decreasing vascular resistance to blood flow. As stated earlier, reducing afterload decreases ventricular wall stress and can improve ventricular performance. Cardiac output will increase, resulting in an improvement of congestion. The combination of diuretics, venodilators, and arterial vasodilators can result in marked improvement in ventricular performance in many patients with decompensated congestive heart failure.

Inotropic Support

In severely decompensated heart failure associated with hypotension and renal insufficiency, aggressive use of diuretics and vasodilators may be quite difficult. Attempts to rapidly achieve high doses of angiotensin-converting enzyme (ACE) inhibitors or adequate doses of β-blockers may also worsen the clinical situation. These very ill patients depend on the activation of the adrenergic and renin–angiotensin–aldosterone systems for life support. Augmenting this support with an intravenous inotropic agent, such as an exogenous catechol (e.g., dobutamine), or a phosphodiesterase inhibitor (milrinone) can increase contractility and cardiac output, resulting in improved renal perfusion and a greater response to diuretic therapy. A period of hemodynamic support with an inotropic agent often promotes some improvement in ventricular geometry, allowing the institution of and rapid up-titration of ACE inhibitors and neurohumoral blockers.

After the inotropic support has been withdrawn and the oral medical program has been stabilized, an assessment of hemodynamic status, including the measurement of right heart pressures and cardiac output, should be performed. A subset of patients will improve clinically but continue to have markedly elevated pulmonary pressures, and a few may have perilously low forward cardiac output.

In a series of patients treated with inotropic-supported up-titration of ACE inhibitor therapy who were then subsequently followed as potential transplant recipients, we found that elevations in pulmonary vascular resistance responded to medical reduction of MR, as well as to surgical reductions. The manipulation of LV loading conditions that can be accomplished with currently available ACE inhibitors; angiotensin-receptor blockers; direct-acting vasodilators; and rate-control agents, including β-blockers, amiodarone, and AV nodal ablation with rate-responsive pacing, is truly remarkable. With patience, slow titration, and inotropic support, the vast majority of heart failure patients can enjoy effective palliation of their symptoms.

SUMMARY

The neurohumoral response to heart failure and the hemodynamic alterations of the disease state are intimately related manifestations of the pathophysiologic process, not separate therapeutic issues. The primary care physician who grasps the essence of this analysis will quickly see the logic of vigorous afterload reduction with ACE inhibitors, control of excessive sympathetic tone with judicious β-adrenergic blockade, and the minimal use of diuretics to avoid intravascular volume depletion and further stimulation of the neurohumoral mechanisms activated by low forward cardiac output.

REFERENCES

1. Braunwald E, Ross J Jr, Sonnenblick EH. Mechanisms of contraction of the normal and failing heart, 2nd ed. Boston: Little, Brown, 1976.
2. Stevenson LW, Miller L. Cardiac transplantation as therapy for heart failure. Curr Probl Cardiol 1991;16:219–305.
3. Stevenson LW. Tailored therapy before transplantation for treatment of advanced heart failure: effective use of vasodilators and diuretics. J Heart Lung Transplant 1991;10:468–476.
4. Stevenson LW, Brunken RC, Belil D, et al. Afterload reduction with vasodilators and diuretics decreases mitral regurgitation during upright exercise in advanced heart failure. J Am Coll Cardiol 1990;15:174–180.
5. Konstam MA, Cohen SR, Salem DN, et al. Comparison of left and right ventricular end-systolic pressure-volume relations in congestive heart failure. J Am Coll Cardiol 1985;5:1326–1334.

SUGGESTED READING

Armstrong PW, Moe CW. Medical advances in the treatment of congestive heart failure. Circulation 1993;88:2941–2952.

Hamilton MA, Stevenson LW, Child JS, et al. Acute reduction of atrial overload during vasodilator and diuretic therapy in advanced congestive heart failure. Am J Cardiol 1990;65:1209–1212.

LeJemtel TH, Demopuolos L, Testa M, Galvao M. Practical aspects of intravenous inotropic therapy for the management of acute and chronic heart failure. Congestive Heart Failure 1995;1:26–29.

Weiland DS, Konstam MA, Salem DN, et al. Contribution of reduced mitral regurgitant volume to vasodilator effect in severe left ventricular failure secondary to coronary artery disease or idiopathic dilated cardiomyopathy. Am J Cardiol 1986;58:1046–1050.

Chapter 5

Clinical Trials That Have Shaped Heart Failure Treatment Protocols

James B. Young

Treatment for heart failure has changed dramatically over the past two decades. Large, carefully designed, and appropriately controlled clinical trials (often with mortality end points) have served practitioners well by providing the objective information that now shapes our practice of evidence-based medicine. Evidence-based medicine is the use of clinical trial experience to make decisions regarding the day-to-day care of individual patients. Table 5.1 details how evidence-based medical practice evolves in general terms. First, the everyday encounters with clinical patients present therapeutic challenges and raise important questions. Basic research tests the treatment hypotheses and leads to the rational design of clinical trials, which should provide more nearly conclusive results. Treatment strategies based on the clinical trials begin to emerge. Appropriate protocols can be developed and practice patterns altered when the treatment strategies have been tested. Adherence to these protocols eventually provides one measure of clinical practice quality.

Table 5.2 summarizes why clinical trials serve as substrate for evidence-based clinical practice. Clinical trials can establish reasonable treatment algorithms and uncover detrimental practices, an issue that is emphasized here. These studies can also determine both the cost of intervention and the cost savings generated by specific therapeutic strategies. Clinical trials are the best, though certainly not the only, means of creating care standards.

Important issues for evaluating results from a clinical trial are summarized in Table 5.3. Specific hypotheses and patient selection

Table 5.1.   Evolution of Evidence-Based Medical Practice

Clinical experience defines therapeutic challenges
• Observations of treatment needed
• Therapeutic successes and failures needed
Research and experimentation
• Basic science research
• Human and/or animal models
• Clinical trial implementation
Clinical treatment strategies designed
• Translation of clinical trial results into clinical practice
• Therapeutic algorithms and protocols instituted
Education
• Caregivers are taught clinical algorithms
• Patients are informed about treatment expectations
Implementation
• Clinical practice patterns influenced
Assessment of strategies
• Analysis of outcomes
• Accountability (adherence to protocol; quality assurance)
• Redefinition of new therapeutic challenges

Table 5.2.   Clinical Trials in Medicine

• Confirm hypotheses regarding therapeutic interventions
• Establish treatment algorithms
• Uncover detrimental routine clinical practices
• Allow more precise risk:benefit calculation for treatment options
• Quantify treatment cost and cost savings engendered by various interventions
• Create care standards for quality assessments

criteria should be stated. The report should explain not only why certain groups were included in the clinical trial but also why exclusions occurred. Sample sizes must be large enough so that statistically meaningful conclusions can be reached. Treatment regimens must be well defined, bias controlled, and random so that comparative groups are similar. End points must be carefully chosen, appropriate to the condition being studied, and well characterized. Acceptable statistical power should be prestated so that the confidence limits of observations are understood. Finally, appropriate procedures for handling clinical trial dropouts, drop-ins, and patients lost to follow-up need to be considered.

Table 5.3.   Issues to Consider When Evaluating a Clinical Trial Report

- Is the hypothesis clearly stated and understood?
- Have patient selection criteria been precisely defined?
- What about characterization of patients not studied?
- Are sample sizes reasonable?
- Were therapeutic and ancillary treatment regimens well defined?
- Are bias controls presented and justified?
- Has randomization been ensured?
- Are end points appropriate and well characterized?
- Have α and β error levels been prestated?
- What were the procedures for handling dropouts, drop-ins, and lost-to-follow-up subjects?

REVIEW OF CLINICAL HEART FAILURE TRIALS

This section discusses clinical trials that have been important to the broad spectrum of heart failure (1–41). The trials are summarized in Table 5.4, where they are ordered alphabetically according to acronym (or short name) rather than in historic sequence. As an overview, these landmark clinical studies, beginning in the late 1970s, generally focused on pharmaceutical strategies, but a few evaluated surgical interventions as well. Several inotropic agents with varying degrees of vasodilating properties improved heart failure symptoms at the cost of higher death rates. Many antiarrhythmic agents were detrimental in heart failure or left ventricular dysfunction (LVD), even though heart failure patients frequently die of malignant ventricular arrhythmias. Calcium channel blockers produced more problems than benefit.

More specifically, the first large-scale mortality end point clinical trial in heart failure was the initial Veterans Administration Cooperative Study of Vasodilator Heart Failure Trial (VeHEFT-I). This study of 642 males with moderate congestive heart failure (CHF) was a pivotal trial because it was the first to suggest that vasodilators beneficially affected mortality in CHF patients. This controversial hypothesis was, to many, disconcerting. The hypothesis speculated that lowered impedance to left ventricular ejection with subsequent reduction of blood pressure and augmentation of forward flow could be translated into improvement in symptoms, better ventricular function, and lower mortality.

Table 5.4. Clinical Trials with Relevance to Managing Patients with Heart Failure

Trial Name	Design and Mean Follow-Up	End Points	Intervention	Number of Patients, Mean Age, Ejection Fraction	Results	Reference
Acute Infarction Ramipril Evaluation (AIRE)	• Placebo controlled • Randomized • Double-blind • Parallel • Multicenter • Post-MI, clinical CHF • 15-month FU	• Total mortality • Development of CHF • Reinfarction • Stroke	Ramipril, 2.5–5 mg bid	• 1,986 • 65 years • NA	• Lower mortality with ramipril (17%) than with placebo (23%) • Mortality reduction apparent at 30 days postinfarct • ACE inhibitor beneficial in patient with clinical CHF after MI	1
Australia-New Zealand Collaborative Carvedilol Trial (AUS-NZ Carvedilol)	• Placebo controlled • Randomized • Double-blind • Parallel • Multicenter • CAD patients • 6-month FU	• EF and treadmill exercise time and distance • LV size • 6-min walk • CHF symptoms and use of drugs	Carvedilol, 3.125 mg qd titrated to 25 mg bid	• 442 • 67 years • 28% EF	• LVEF up 5.2% ($p < .0001$) • LV size down • No change in ETT • No change in 6-min walk • Symptoms largely unchanged	2
Canadian Myocardial Infarction Amiodarone Trial (CAMIAT)	• Placebo controlled • Randomized • Double-blind • Parallel	• Resuscitated Vfib • Arrhythmic death	Amiodarone: 10 mg/kg × 2 weeks 400 mg × 2 weeks 300 mg × 12 weeks	• 1,202 • 64 years • NA	• Resuscitated Vfib/ arrhythmic death down (RR = 49%; $p = .016$)	3

Study	Methods/Design	Endpoints	Drug/Dose	Patients	Outcomes	Ref
	• Multicenter • Post-MI • 22-month FU	• Other cardiac death • Noncardiac vascular death	200 mg qd		• All cause mortality not reduced • 36% of amiodarone group stopped drug compared to placebo	
U.S. Carvedilol Heart Failure Study Group (Carvedilol-Combined USA)	• Pooled data from Carvedilol-MOCHA, -PRECISE, -Mild CHF, and -Severe CHF • 7-month FU	• Total mortality (obtained as safety issue) • Hospitalizations	Carvedilol, 3.125–25 mg bid	• 1,098 • 58 years • 23% EF	• Mortality down by 65% ($p < .001$) • Hospitalizations down by 27% ($p = .036$) • Combined death/hospitalization down ($p < .001$)	4
U.S. Carvedilol Heart Failure Study Group (Carvedilol-Mild CHF)	• Placebo controlled • Randomized • Double-blind • Parallel • Multicenter • 12-month FU	• Clinically worse CHF; death, hospitalization, more meds • ΔEF • QOL; NYHA class; CHF self-assessment • 6-min walk	Carvedilol, 3.125–25 mg bid	• 366 • 54 years • 23% EF	• Progression of CHF down by 48% ($p = .008$) • No change in walk or QOL	5
Multicenter Oral Carvedilol Assessment (Carvedilol-MOCHA)	• Placebo controlled • Randomized • Double-blind • Parallel • Multicenter • Dose ranging • 6-min walk base = 450–550 M	• Submaximal exercise • CHF self-assessment • QOL • NYHA Class • ΔEF • Mortality/	Carvedilol, 6.25, 12.5, 25 mg bid	• 345 • 60 years • 23% EF	• No change in exercise • EF up by 5, 6, and 8% for these doses ($p < .001$) • Mortality down by 73% ($p < .001$) • Hospitalization down ($p = 0.1$)	6

(continued)

Table 5.4. (*Continued*)

Trial Name	Design and Mean Follow-Up	End Points	Intervention	Number of Patients, Mean Age, Ejection Fraction	Results	Reference
	• 12-month FU	hospitalization (as safety issue)				
Randomized Prospective Evaluation of Carvedilol on Symptoms and Exercise Trial (Carvedilol-PRECISE)	• Placebo controlled • Double-blind • Parallel • Multicenter • 6-min walk base = 150–450 M • 6-month FU	• Submaximal exercise • CHF self-assessment • QOL • NYHA Class • ΔEF • Mortality/ hospitalization (as safety issue)	Carvedilol, 6.25–25 mg bid	• 277 • 60 years • 22% EF	• No change in exercise • No change in QOL • Improved NYHA class, global assessment • EF up ($p = .001$) • Mortality/ hospitalization down ($p = .029$)	7
Cardiac Arrhythmia Suppression Trial (CAST)	• Placebo controlled • Randomized • Double-blind • Multicenter • Post-MI with mildly symptomatic ventricular arrhythmia • 10-month FU	• Arrhythmic death • Total mortality	Encainmide, flecainmide, or moricizine titrated to arrhythmia control	• 2,309 • 61 years • 40% EF (48% with EF < 40%)	• Mortality with encainmide and flecainmide up • RR up 2.5 ($p < .001$) • Class 1C antiarrhythmic drugs likely detrimental in patients post-MI with heart failure	8

Study	Design	Endpoints	Intervention	Characteristics	Results	
Cardiac Arrhythmia Suppression Trial II (CAST II)	• Placebo controlled • Randomized • Double-blind • Parallel • Multicenter • EF < 40% post-MI with mildly symptomatic ventricular arrhythmia • 18-month FU	• Total mortality	Moricizine, 600–900 mg qd (based on arrhythmia control)	• 1,325 • 62 years • 32% EF	• Stopped early secondary excess mortality with moricizine in first 2 weeks post-MI (proarrhythmia)	9
Congestive Heart Failure Survival Trial of Amiodarone Therapy (CHF-STAT)	• Placebo controlled • Double-blind • Parallel • Multicenter • 45-month FU	• Total mortality • SCD syndrome • ΔEF • VT suppression	Amiodarone: 800 mg × 14 days 400 mg × 50 weeks 300 mg qd	• 674 • 65 years • 66% EF • <30% EF	• No change in mortality ($p = .6$) • No change in SCD ($p = .43$) • EF up ($p < .001$) • Trend toward lower mortality in nonischemic group ($p = .07$) • 27% of amiodarone group stopped drug	10
Cardiac Insufficiency Bisoprolol Study (CIBIS Trial)	• Placebo controlled • Randomized • Double-blind • Multicenter • Mild to moderate heart failure • 23-month FU	• Total mortality	Bisoprolol, 1.25–5.0 mg/day	• 641 • 59 years • 25% EF	• Mortality down by 20% ($p = .22$) • Improved LV function • Heart failure hospitalizations down • Mortality benefit noted in patients without prior MI	11

(continued)

Table 5.4. (*Continued*)

Trial Name	Design and Mean Follow-Up	End Points	Intervention	Number of Patients, Mean Age, Ejection Fraction	Results	Reference
Cooperative North Scandanavian Enalapril Survival Study (CONSENSUS)	• Placebo controlled • Randomized • Double-blind • Parallel • Multicenter • Class IV CHF • 6-month FU	• Total mortality • Cardiac mortality	Enalapril, 5–10 mg bid	• 253 • 70 years • NA	• Mortality down by 40% ($p = .002$) • Heart size down • Improved NYHA class • No effect on SCD	12
Digitalis investigation Group (DIG)	• Placebo controlled • Randomized • Double-blind • Parallel • Multicenter • Included diastolic dysfunction • 37-month FU	• Total mortality • Hospitalization for CHF • QOL	Digoxin, 0.125–0.5 mg (based on weight/creatinine algorithm)	• 7,788 • 64 years • 32% EF	• No change in mortality • Hospitalization down by 37% ($p < .001$) • Little digoxin toxicity	13
Evaluation of Losartan in the Elderly Study (ELITE)	• Captopril controlled • Randomized • Double-blind • Parallel • Multicenter • 12-month FU	• Development of renal dysfunction • Combined mortality/hospitalization • Total mortality	Losartan, 50 mg vs. captopril 50 mg tid	• 722 • 74 years • 31% EF	• No change in renal function • Mortality/hospitalization down (RR = 0.075) • Mortality down by 46% ($p = .32$)	14

Study	Design	Drug	Outcomes	Patients	Results	
European Myocardial Infarction Amiodarone Trial (EMIAT)	• Placebo controlled • Randomized • Double-blind • Parallel • Multicenter • 21-month FU	Amiodarone 800 mg × 14 days 400 mg × 14 weeks 200 mg qd	• Total mortality • Cardiac mortality and arrhythmic death	• 1,486 • 60 years • 30% EF	• No change in total mortality • Arrhythmic deaths down by 35% ($p = .05$) • 39% of amiodarone group stopped drug	15
Flosequinan-ACE Inhibitor Trial (FACET)	• Placebo controlled • Randomized • Double-blind • Parallel • Multicenter • 4-month FU	Flosequinan, 100 mg qd or 75 mg bid	• Exercise tolerance • QOL	• 322 • 58 years • 23% EF	• 100 mg qd improved exercise time • QOL improved • Headache, palpitations, tachycardia seen as side effects	16
Grupo de Estudio de la Sobrevida en la Insuficiencia Cardiaca en Argentina [Group Study of Heart Failure in Argentina] (GESICA)	• Placebo controlled • Randomized • Unblinded • Parallel • Multicenter • Dilated or CAD heart failure • 13-month FU	Amiodarone: 600 mg dq × 4 days 300 mg qd	• Total mortality • Subgroup mortality • SCD vs. CHF death • CHF hospitalizations	• 516 • 59 years • 20% EF	• Total mortality down by 28% ($p = .024$) • SCD and CHF mortality reduction similar • Death/hospitalization down by 31% ($p = .002$) • Amiodarone associated with frequent side effects	17
Gruppo Italiano per lo Studio della Supravvivenza nell-Infarto Miocardio	• Placebo controlled • Randomized • Double-blind • Parallel	Lisinopril: 5–10 mg qd TNG patch 10 mg qd	• Total mortality • ΔEF	• 18,895 • NA • NA	• Mortality down by 11% with lisinopril ($p = .001$) • No change with TNF	18

(continued)

Table 5.4. (*Continued*)

Trial Name	Design and Mean Follow-Up	End Points	Intervention	Number of Patients, Mean Age, Ejection Fraction	Results	Reference
[Effect of Transdermal TNG and Lisinopril on Postinfarction Survival] (GISSI-3)	• Multicenter • Routine post-MI therapy • 1.5-month FU					
International Study of Infarct Survival (ISIS-IV)	• Placebo controlled • Randomized • Double-blind • Parallel • Multicenter • Routine post-MI therapy • 1-month FU	• Total mortality • Development of CHF	Captopril, 6.25–50 mg bid Imdur: 30–60 mg qd iv Mg^{2+} acutely	• 58,050 • NA • NA	• Mortality down by 7% with captopril ($p = .02$) • Mg^{2+} and oral mononitrate had no impact	19
Multicenter Automatic Defibrillator Implantation Trial (MADIT)	• Antiarrhythmic drug controlled • Randomized • Parallel • Multicenter • Post-MI with malignant ventricular arrhythmia • 27-month FU	• Total mortality • Arrhythmic death • Nonarrhythmic death	AICD vs. best medical therapy	• 253 • 63 years • 26% EF	• Mortality down with AICD ($p = .009$)	20

Trial	Design	Outcomes	Intervention	Characteristics	Results	Ref
Metoprolol in Dilated Cardiomyopathy Trial (MDC)	• Placebo controlled • Randomized • Double-blind • Parallel • Multicenter • Dilated cardiomyopathy only • 12-month FU	• Death/Htx listing • ΔEF • CHF symptoms	Metoprolol, 10 to 100–150 mg qd	• 383 • NA • 100% EF < 40% EF	• Symptoms improved • EF up • Exercise time greater • Less need for Htx • No change in mortality	21
Multicenter Diltiazem Post Infarction Trial (MDPIT)	• Placebo controlled • Randomized • Double-blind • Parallel • Multicenter • Post-MI (early) • 25-month FU	• Total mortality • Cardiac death • Nonfatal MI	Diltiazem, 60 mg bid, qid	• 2,466 • 58 years • 46% EF	• No mortality change overall • More cardiac events with diltiazem when EF < 40% • When EF < 40% 21% on diltiazem developed clinical CHF vs. 12% on placebo	22
Myocarditis Treatment Trial (Myocarditis)	• Placebo controlled • Randomized • Double-blind • Parallel • Multicenter • 7-month FU	• ΔEF at 28 weeks • Mortality or heart transplant • Change in endomyocardial biopsy	Cyclosporine, prednisone, azathioprine vs. standard therapy	• 111 • 42 years • 25% EF	• No change in EF by therapy • No survival advantage with immunosuppression	23
Pimobendan in Congestive Heart Failure (PICO)	• Placebo controlled • Randomized • Double-blind	• Exercise time • NYHA class • QOL	Pimobendan, 25–50 mg qd	• 317 • 65 years • 27% EF	• Exercise times up • No change in VO_2max or QOL	24

(continued)

Table 5.4. (Continued)

Trial Name	Design and Mean Follow-Up	End Points	Intervention	Number of Patients, Mean Age, Ejection Fraction	Results	Reference
Prospective Randomized Amlodipine Survival Evaluation (PRAISE)	• Placebo controlled • Randomized • Double-blind • Parallel • Multicenter • 14-month FU	• Combined total mortality/CV mortality • Total mortality	Amlodipine, 10 mg qd	• 1,153 • 64 years • 21% EF	• Death hazard up with Pimobendan (1.8; 95% CI 0.9–3.5) • No change in combined mortality/morbidity end point • Mortality down by 16% ($p = .07$) • Primary end point down in nonischemic group • Amlodipine reasonably well tolerated	25
Prospective Randomized Study of Ibopamine on Mortality and Efficacy (PRIME II)	• Placebo controlled • Randomized • Double-blind • Parallel • Multicenter • 12-month FU	• Total mortality • Cardiac mortality • Hospitalization • Symptoms	Ibopamine, 300 mg qd	• 1,906 • 65 years • 20% EF	• Mortality up in the ibopamine group (RR = 1.26; $p = .017$)	26
Prospective Randomized Flosequinan Longevity	• Placebo controlled • Randomized • Double-blind • Parallel	• Total mortality • CHF hospitalization	Flosequinan, 75 or 100 mg qd	• 2,304 • NA • 100% EF < 35% EF	• Mortality up (RR = 1.43; $p < .05$) • CHF hospitalizations up	27

Study	Design	Intervention	Patients	Outcomes	Results	Ref
Evaluation (PROFILE)	• Multicenter • 22-month FU				• Study forced flosequinan from market	
Prospective Randomized Milrinone Survival Evaluation (PROMISE)	• Placebo controlled • Randomized • Double-blind • Parallel • Multicenter • 6-month FU	Milrinone, 40 mg/day	• 1,088 • 64 years • 21% EF	• Total mortality • Cardiac mortality • CHF hospitalization • Adverse reactions	• Mortality up by 28% ($p = .038$) • Cardiac mortality up by 34% ($p = .016$) • Adverse mortality effect greatest in most ill patients	28
Prospective Randomized Study of Ventricular Failure and the Efficacy of Digoxin (PROVED)	• Placebo controlled • Randomized • Double-blind • Parallel • Multicenter • Digoxin withdrawal on background of diuretic 3-month FU	Digoxin, 0.125–0.5 mg qd (based on weight/creatinine algorithm)	• 88 • 64 years • 28% EF	• Exercise tolerance • ΔEF • CHF	• Digoxin withdrawal caused worse heart failure	29
Randomized Digoxin and Inhibitor of Angiotensin-Converting Enzyme Inhibitor Trial (RADIANCE)	• 3-month FU • Placebo controlled • Randomized • Double-blind • Parallel • Multicenter • Digoxin withdrawal on background of	Digoxin, 0.125–0.5 mg qd (based on weight/creatine algorithm)	• 178 • 60 years • 27% EF	• Exercise tolerance • ΔEF • CHF symptoms	• Digoxin withdrawal caused worse heart failure	30

(continued)

Table 5.4. (*Continued*)

Trial Name	Design and Mean Follow-Up	End Points	Intervention	Number of Patients, Mean Age, Ejection Fraction	Results	Reference
Survival and Ventricular Enlargement Trial (SAVE)	diuretic/ACE inhibitor • 3-month FU • Placebo controlled • Randomized • Double-blind • Parallel • Multicenter • Post-MI with EF < 40% (early) • 42-month FU	• Total mortality • Cardiac mortality • ΔEF	Captopril, 25–50 mg tid	• 2,231 • 59 years • 31% EF	• Mortality down by 19% ($p = .019$) • CHF down by 37% ($p < .001$) • MI down by 25% ($p = .015$)	31
Survival of Myocardial Infarction Long-Term Evaluation Study (SMILE)	• Placebo controlled • Randomized • Double-blind • Parallel • Multicenter • 1.5-month FU	• Death or worse CHF • 1 year mortality	Zofenopril, 30 mg qd	• 1,556 • 64 years • 28% EF	• Mortality/CHF down by 34% at 6 weeks ($p = 0.18$) • Mortality at 1 year down by 29% ($p = .011$)	32
Studies of Left Ventricular Dysfunction Trial—Prevention (SOLVD-	• Placebo controlled • Randomized • Double-blind • Parallel • Multicenter	• Total mortality • Hospitalization • Morbidity	Enalapril, 2.5–10 mg bid	• 4,228 • 59 years • 25% EF	• Mortality down by 16% ($p < .001$) • Death/CHF hospitalization down by 26% ($p < .001$)	33

Trial	Design	Treatment	Endpoints	Patient characteristics	Results	Ref
Prevention)	• Class I–II LVD • 37-month FU				• No SCD reduction	
Studies of Left Ventricular Dysfunction Trial—Treatment (SOLVD-Treatment)	• Placebo controlled • Randomized • Double-blind • Parallel • Multicenter • Class II–III CHF • 41-month FU	Enalapril, 2.5–10 mg bid	• Total mortality • Hospitalization • Morbidity	• 2,569 • 61 years • 28% EF	• Mortality down by 8% (p = .3) • Death/CHF hospitalization down by 29% (p < .001) • CHF hospitalization down by 36% (p = .001)	34
Survival with Oral d-Sotolol Trial (SWORD)	• Placebo controlled • Randomized • Double-blind • Parallel • Multicenter • 28-month FU	d-Sotolol, 100–200 mg bid	• Total mortality • Cardiac mortality • Arrhythmic death • Arrhythmic event • Hospitalization	• 3,121 • 60 years • 31% EF	• Mortality down with Sotolol (RR = 1.65, p = .006) • Arrhythmic deaths down (RR = 1.77) • Adverse outcome greater in lower EF patients	35
Trandolapril Cardiac Evaluation Trial (TRACE)	• Placebo controlled • Randomized • Double-blind • Parallel • Multicenter • 6-month FU	Trandolapril, 1 mg qd	• Total mortality • Cardiovascular mortality	• 1,749 • 67 years • NA	• Mortality down with trandolapril (RR = 78; p = .001) • CHF down (RR = .071; p = .003)	36
Vesnarinone Study Group (Vesnarinone)	• Placebo controlled • Randomized • Double-blind • Parallel • Multicenter	Vesnarinone, 60 or 120 mg qd	• Cardiovascular morbidity/ mortality (morbidity = CHF hospital	• 477 • 56 years • 20% EF	• 120 mg dosing stopped secondary mortality rise • 60 mg lowered morbidity/mortality	37

(continued)

Table 5.4. (*Continued*)

Trial Name	Design and Mean Follow-Up	End Points	Intervention	Number of Patients, Mean Age, Ejection Fraction	Results	Reference
	• Class I–IV CHF • 6-month FU	admit for inotrope) • Total mortality			by 50% ($p = .003$) • 60 mg lowered total mortality by 62% ($p = .008$) • 2.5% incidence of neutropenia noted • VEST showed rise in mortality with 60 and 30 mg doses	
Veterans Administration Cooperative Study of Vasodilator Heart Failure Trial (VeHEFT-I)	• Placebo controlled • Randomized • Double-blind • Parallel • Multicenter • Class II–III CHF • 28-month FU	• Total mortality • ΔEF	Hydralazine, 300 mg qd Isosorbide dinitrate, 160 mg qd Prazosin, 20 mg qd	• 642 • 58 years • 30% EF	• Hydralazine/isosorbide dinitrate lowered mortality by 34% ($p = .028$) • No benefit with prazosin • EF up with hydralazine/isosorbide dinitrate	38
Veterans Administration Cooperative Study of Vasodilator Heart	• Active drug (HYD/ISDN) controlled • Randomized	• Total mortality • ΔEF • CHF symptoms	Enalapril, 10 mg bid Hydralazine, 300 mg qd Isosorbide dinitrate, 160 mg qd	• 804 • 60 years • 29% EF	• Enalapril lowered mortality more by 18% ($p = .016$); hydralazine/	39

Study	Design	End points	Drug/dose	Patients	Results	Ref
Failure Trial II (VeHEFT-II)	• Double-blind • Parallel • Multicenter • Class II–III CHF • 30-month FU				isosorbide dinitrate by 25% • HYD/ISDN ↑ EF more • Hydralazine/isosorbine dinitrate increased EF more than enalapril did	40
Veterans Administration Cooperative Study of Vasodilator Heart Failure Trial III (VeHEFT-III)	• Placebo controlled • Randomized • Double-blind • Parallel • Multicenter • Class II-III CHF • 36-month FU	• Exercise tolerance • Morbidity • Total mortality	Felodipine, 2.5–5 mg bid	• 451 • 63 years • 30% EF	• No benefit with felodipine • No complications	
Xamoterol in Severe Heart Failure Study (Xamoterol)	• Placebo controlled • Randomized • Double-blind • Parallel • Multicenter • Class III-IV CHF • 3-month FU	• Exercise tolerance • CHF symptoms • Adverse events	Xamoterol, 200 mg bid	• 516 • 62 years • 25% EF	• No improvements in CHF symptoms • Greater mortality with xamoterol	41

AICD, automatic implantable defibrillating device; *CAD*, coronary artery disease; *CHF*, congestive heart failure; *CI*, confidence interval; *CV*, cardiovascular; *EF*, ejection fraction; *FU*, follow-up; *HTx*, heart transplant; *LV*, left ventricle; *LVD*, left ventricle dysfunction; *LVEF*, left ventricle ejection fraction; *MI*, myocardial infarction; *NA*, not available; *NYHA*, New York Heart Association; *QOL*, quality of life; *RR*, relative risk (>0, increased; <0, decreased); *SCD*, sudden cardiac death; *Vfib*, ventricular fibrillation; *VT*, ventricular tachycardia.

CONSENSUS demonstrated a profound reduction in mortality in severely ill New York Heart Association (NYHA) class IV CHF patients. The reduction in mortality when enalapril was added to digoxin and diuretics supported a new so-called neurohumoral interdiction hypothesis, which speculated that clinical benefit could be achieved by blocking neurohumoral compensatory systems.

Subsequently, the second VeHEFT trial (VeHEFT-II) compared the combination of hydralazine and isosorbide dinitrate (the winning drug combination in VeHEFT-I) to the angiotensin-converting enzyme (ACE) inhibitor enalapril to study the "hemodynamic hypothesis" versus the so-called neurohormonal interdiction hypothesis in heart failure treatment. Enalapril resulted in a greater mortality reduction than did the direct-acting vasodilator combination, although hydralazine and isosorbide dinitrate improved ejection fraction substantially more.

Studies with calcium antagonists generally have demonstrated increased morbidity and mortality in heart failure cohorts. PRAISE and VeHEFT-III are the only clinical trials to date that suggest that the specific calcium channel blocking agents amlodipine and felodipine might not carry such concerns for CHF patients.

The SOLVD Trials examined enalapril in patients who were asymptomatic or only minimally symptomatic (the Prevention Trial) and in patients with mild to moderate congestive heart failure (the Treatment Trial). Baseline, or first-line, medications in the Treatment Trial were diuretics and digoxin; in the Prevention Trial, enalapril was the first-line therapy for asymptomatic left ventricular systolic dysfunction. In patients with an ejection fraction less than 35% (an entry criterion for both trials) and symptomatic heart failure, enalapril significantly reduced mortality; morbidity; and, it is important to note, major ischemic events, such as acute myocardial infarction and hospital admissions for unstable angina during long-term follow-up. These trials suggested that ACE inhibitors attenuated major ischemic events. In fact, there was a more impressive reduction in major ischemic events than in any other single end point, including hospitalization for heart failure, in these trials.

SOLVD-Prevention demonstrated a significant decrement in the combined end point of congestive heart failure morbidity (hospital admissions for worsening CHF) and mortality. This landmark study suggested that a preventive strategy with an ACE inhibitor (enalapril) could attenuate progression to clinical heart failure when used as a first-line therapy in asymptomatic or minimally symptomatic patients with LVD; and in fact, the SOLVD Trials brought about a paradigm shift in the treatment of heart failure.

The massive DIG Trial studied 7788 patients with clinically symptomatic congestive heart. At the 5-year follow-up the study suggested that digoxin did not have a significant impact on mortality but did reduce worsening heart failure defined by hospitalization. A large component of this trial independently confirmed the observations made in the PROVED and RADIANCE Trials that withdrawal of digoxin in clinically stable congestive heart failure patients was associated with worsening heart failure symptoms. All three of these trials support the contention that triple therapy (diuretic, digoxin, and ACE inhibitor) is the best strategy in CHF patients.

The SAVE Trial demonstrated improved survival and functional status and reduced repeat myocardial infarction (MI) rate with captopril in acute MI patients who had a postinfarct ejection fraction less than 40%. Therapy was begun within the 1st week after myocardial infarction. Other clinical trials—including AIRE, SMILE, and TRACE—have confirmed that ACE inhibitors begun shortly after myocardial infarction have significant benefits for patients with either asymptomatic left ventricular systolic dysfunction or mild clinical heart failure. Captopril, ramipril, zofenopril, and trandolapril have positive results, suggesting a class effect of ACE inhibitors. Several megatrials with ACE inhibitors also confirm that therapy after myocardial infarction reduces short-term mortality. The fourth International Study of Infarct Survival (ISIS-IV) Trial and the third Gruppo Italieno per lo Studio della Sopravvivenza Infarto Miocardio (GISSI-3) Trial included patients with a wide spectrum of ejection fractions; their findings suggest that early administration of captopril or lisinopril translates into postinfarction benefit.

Use of β-adrenergic blocking drugs has been the focus of several clinical trials in heart failure patients over the last decade. The MDC study compared the β_1-selective β-blocker metoprolol to placebo prescribed in addition to background heart failure therapy for dilated cardiomyopathy. Patients in the active treatment limb had improved symptoms with a reduction in the combined end point of survival and need for cardiac transplantation. Subsidiary end points such as ejection fraction and heart failure symptoms were also beneficially affected by metoprolol. More recently, the Carvedilol-PRECISE and the Carvedilol-MOCHA Trials demonstrated improvement in mild to moderate heart failure patients receiving this β-blocker–vasodilator compound in addition to digoxin, diuretics, and ACE inhibitors.

A pooled analysis of four large carvedilol treatment protocols (Carvedilol-Combined USA) implied that mortality was reduced substantially. Though the data were intriguing, the studies were not primarily mortality end point driven clinical trials. Exercise tolerance generally did not improve with carvedilol; subjective assessments such as heart failure functional class and global assessment of clinical heart failure profiles did improve, as did ejection fraction. The results of these trials, in conjunction with observations made in the AUS-NZ Carvedilol Trial, suggest that carvedilol, a β-adrenergic blocking compound with α-adrenergic blocking activity, will play a major role in therapy for mild to moderate heart failure. Dose-titration protocols similar to those used in the clinical trials should be standard practice.

Malignant ventricular arrhythmias are frequent and devastating in patients with systolic left ventricular dysfunction and heart failure, but antiarrhythmic drugs have not fared well in clinical trials. The Cardiac Arrhythmia Suppression Trial (CAST) studied encainide, flecainide, and moricizine in post–myocardial infarction patients with multiple premature ventricular contractions and LVD. The patients involved in the encainide and flecainide trial (CAST-I) and in the moricizine trial (CAST-II) resembled those randomized into the SAVE, AIRE, SMILE, and TRACE Trials. CAST-I and CAST-II were terminated prematurely because of excessive mortality in all antiarrhythmic treatment groups. More recently, the SWORD Trial evaluated the effect of d-sotalol on mortality in patients with an ejection fraction less than 40% after myocardial infarction. This trial was also stopped prematurely because of excessive treatment group mortality.

Amiodarone may be the one beneficial antiarrhythmic drug in heart failure. The GESICA Trial was an unblinded, placebo-controlled, mortality end point evaluation of amiodarone in moderate to severe heart failure. Mortality was significantly reduced in the amiodarone group, suggesting that amiodarone could be used safely in CHF patients and might even provide benefit. The drug, however, was stopped frequently by both patients and physicians because of troublesome side effects and pharmacologic toxicity. The unblinded nature of this trial has raised concern regarding the power of the conclusion. EMIAT randomized patients with ejection fractions less than 40% at 5 to 21 days post-MI. Mortality, the primary end point, was not reduced. However, a combined end point of presumed arrhythmic death and resuscitated cardiac arrest diminished slightly.

CAMIAT evaluated patients 6 to 45 days post-MI. The end point was a combination of arrhythmic death and/or resuscitated ventricular fibrillation; all-cause mortality and cardiac mortality were secondary end points. Amiodarone reduced the incidence of ventricular fibrillation and arrhythmic death, but 42% of the treatment group stopped the drug by the 2nd year follow-up point because of toxicity. Both CAMIAT and EMIAT have been criticized for drawing conclusions from end points such as "presumed" ventricular arrhythmic death.

CHF-STAT studied heart failure patients who had at least 10 premature ventricular contractions per hour on ambulatory monitoring; amiodarone did not improve survival compared to placebo. Although the data do not support prophylactic therapy, these trials do not suggest that amiodarone increased mortality. For heart failure patients requiring antiarrhythmic therapy for specific indications, amiodarone remains a reasonable choice.

MADIT evaluated the prophylactic use of an implanted cardioverter defibrillation device compared to conventional medical therapy in patients with prior infarction, with a left ventricular ejection fraction less than 35%, and at high risk for ventricular arrhythmias (defined as asymptomatic, nonsustained ventricular tachycardia with nonsuppressible ventricular tachycardia elicited during electrophysiologic study). Mortality was significantly lower with a device than with conventional antiarrhythmic therapy. This important trial suggests that prophylactic therapy with an automatic implantable cardioverter defibrillating device may be appropriate for selected patients.

Clinical trials with mortality end points have shown that several agents that improve hemodynamics and symptoms in heart failure actually increase death rates. Examples of such studies are PROFILE (flosequinan), PICO (pimobendan), PROMISE (oral milrinone), PRIME II (ibopamine), and the Xamoterol in Severe Heart Failure Study (xamoterol). Milrinone, a potent phosphodiesterase inhibitor with inotropic and vasodilating properties, improved hemodynamics and clinical findings in heart failure patients yet significantly increased mortality caused by sudden cardiac death. Flosequinan, another inotropic vasodilator, provided symptomatic improvement but increased mortality rates. Xamoterol, an agent with intrinsic sympathomimetic activity, has also been shown to increase mortality. Ibopamine, a dopaminergic compound available in Europe, improved symptoms and exercise tolerance but increased mortality, particularly in severe heart failure.

Results with calcium channel blockers in heart failure trials are not encouraging. Although not strictly a heart failure trial, MDPIT demonstrated that diltiazem significantly increased adverse cardiac events in post–myocardial infarction patients with clinically manifest heart failure.

Vesnarinone appears to reduce inflammatory components of the heart failure syndrome. The Vesnarinone Survival Trial (VesT) demonstrated a 24% increase in total mortality with a 60 mg dose of the drug ($p < .05$) and a 12% increase in mortality with a 30 mg dose (p = not significant). An earlier trial by the Vesnarinone Study Group (Vesnarinone) indicated the drug reduced mortality substantially at a 60 mg dose, whereas a 120 mg dose was associated with increased death rates. This set of observations with vesnarinone is still incomplete as data analysis is ongoing, but the disparity between end point effects in two well-designed mortality end point clinical trials is troubling. Perhaps vesnarinone, like other drugs mentioned above, has beneficial effects in only a small subset of patients yet to be characterized.

The Myocarditis Treatment Trial (Myocarditis) studied immunosuppressive therapy in patients with inflammatory heart disease. This trial screened 2233 patients, but enrolled only the 111 patients with biopsy-documented lymphocytic myocarditis. Patients were randomized to evaluate the best heart failure medical care versus cyclosporine or a combination of azathioprine and prednisone. Immunosuppressive therapy was given over 24 weeks; mean follow-up was 7 months, and some patients were followed for 4 years. No differences were found between treatment cohorts. No significant improvement in survival was noted, and there was an extremely high mortality rate overall (20% at 1 year and 56% at 4.3 years). This study suggests no benefit from immunosuppressive therapy in patients with presumed myocarditis.

Finally, the ELITE trial studied losartan in elderly patients with heart failure. The trial was designed to determine whether losartan, a specific angiotensin II receptor–blocking drug, offers safe and efficacious advantages over captopril when given to heart failure patients older than 65 years. The 722 patients were randomized to either captopril (50 mg three times daily) or losartan (50 mg daily) and followed for 1 year. Most patients had NYHA class II disease, and about one-third of the patients had class III disease. The frequency of persistent increases in serum creatinine was the same in both groups. Fewer patients discontinued losartan because of adverse experiences; and no losartan-treated patient stopped the drug for cough, although 12 of 370 captopril patients did so. Death and/or heart failure hospitalization was 9.4% in the losartan patients versus 13.2% in the captopril patients, a risk reduction of 32% ($p = .075$). Losartan decreased all-cause mortality by 46% (4.8% in the losartan group versus 8.7% in the captopril group; $p = .02$). Sudden cardiac death was much less in the losartan group; risk reduction was 64% (95% confidence interval: 0.03–0.86). Losartan was generally better tolerated. ELITE is the first clinical trial to suggest that angiotensin II blockade can reduce heart failure symptoms and mortality. These drugs may offer a viable alternative to ACE inhibitors. It is tantalizing to speculate that these agents might provide greater mortality reduction than ACE inhibitors or provide advantages when combined with them.

SUMMARY

Table 5.5 summarizes what we have learned from two decades of clinical trials focused on heart failure patients. Direct-acting vasodilating drugs may not dramatically decrease mortality, despite improved hemodynamics. Many trials have confirmed the role of ACE inhibitors as the primary option in patients with either asymptomatic LVD or CHF more generally. ACE inhibitors also benefit patients suffering acute myocardial infarction, particularly those with postinfarct left ventricular systolic dysfunction or symptomatic congestive heart failure. Furthermore, trials have shown that angiotensin II blocking compounds may provide an attractive option for heart failure patients experiencing intolerable side effects with ACE inhibitor therapy.

Table 5.5.   What We Have Learned from Heart Failure Clinical Trials

- The treatment paradigm has shifted from diuretic and inotropic–based protocols to ones designed to interdict neurohumoral, humoral, and cytokine activation.
- ACE inhibitors are the first line therapy for heart failure.
- Treatment protocols should begin early in patients with asymptomatic left ventricular systolic dysfunction to prevent deterioration.
- Triple therapy—diuretics, digoxin, and ACE inhibitors—is baseline in congestive heart failure patients.
- Digoxin does not beneficially or adversely affect mortality in heart failure but clearly improves symptomatology.
- The routine prescription of antiarrhythmic therapy in patients with LVD carries substantive risk of increased mortality.
- Amiodarone may be acceptable in heart failure patients when pharmacologic treatment of atrial fibrillation or ventricular arrhythmias is required, but it does not appear to offer significant benefit when routinely prescribed.
- Automatic implantable defibrillating devices may be the preferable approach to complex ventricular arrhythmias in the heart failure setting when associated with symptoms such as syncope or sudden cardiac death syndrome.
- β-adrenergic blocking drugs (especially carvedilol) may be helpful when used as adjunctive therapy with baseline triple drug protocols.
- Not all vasodilators (e.g., dihydropyridine calcium channel blockers) that improve heart failure hemodynamics are associated with lower morbidity and mortality.
- Diagnosis of myocarditis is problematic, and immunosuppressive therapies have not proven beneficial.
- Chronic inotropic therapy seemingly reduces morbidity but increases mortality (with the exception of digoxin).
- ACE inhibitors should be prescribed early after myocardial infarction.
- Angiotensin II receptor blockers may prove to be alternatives in heart failure patients who cannot tolerate ACE inhibitors.

Carvedilol, a β-adrenergic blocking agent with vasodilating properties, has a useful role in mild to moderate heart failure syndromes in addition to digoxin and diuretic therapy. Amiodarone may be the most reasonable option when antiarrhythmic drugs are necessary, although automatic cardioverter defibrillating devices may be the preferred tactic for heart failure complicated by potentially malignant ventricular arrhythmias. Digoxin remains an important drug to prevent morbidity in CHF patients.

The stronger inotropic agents, pimobendan and ibopamine, on the other hand, carry an unacceptable mortality profile, even though these drugs improve symptoms. Likewise, flosequinan, milrinone, and vesnarinone may improve heart failure symptoms, but they increase mortality and, particularly, sudden cardiac death. Although many studies have suggested detrimental results when calcium channel blocking drugs are used, amlodipine and felodipine may be exceptions. These drugs are not associated with increased mortality and morbidity; however, they do not reduce these important end points. If indicated for angina or hypertension, amlodipine and felodipine may be safely added to a standard three-drug heart failure prescription.

Clinical trials have, indeed taught us much with respect to heart failure therapeutics. Ongoing studies of other β-blockers (bucindolol), inotropic agents (levosimendan), calcium channel blockers (mibefradil), atrial natriuretic peptides, and endothelin inhibitors will likely shape future treatment of heart failure patients.

REFERENCES

1. Acute Infarction Ramipril Efficacy Study Investigators. Effect of ramipril on mortality and morbidity of survivors of acute myocardial infarction with clinical evidence of heart failure. Lancet 1993;342:821–828.
2. Australia-New Zealand Heart Failure Research Collaborative Group. Effects of carvedilol in patients with congestive heart failure due to ischemic heart disease: final results from the Australia-New Zealand Heart Failure Research Collaborative Group Trial. Lancet 1997;349:387–390.
3. Cairns JA, Connolly SJ, Roberts R, Gent M. Randomised trial of outcome after myocardial infarction in patients with frequent or repetitive ventricular premature depolarisations: CAMIAT. Canadian Amiodarone Myocardial Infarction Arrhythmia Trial Investigators. Lancet 1997;349:675–682.
4. Packer M, Bristow MR, Cohn JN, et al. The effect of carvedilol on morbidity and mortality in patients with chronic heart failure. Randomized Amlodipine Survival Evaluation Study Group. N Engl J Med 1996;334:1349–1355.
5. Colucci WS, Packer M, Bristow MR, et al. Carvedilol inhibits clinical progression in patients with mild symptoms of heart failure. US Carvedilol Heart Failure Study Group. Circulation 1996;94:2800–2806.
6. Bristow MR, Gilbert EM, Abraham WT, et al. Carvedilol produces dose-related improvements in left ventricular function and survival in subjects with chronic heart failure. MOCHA Investigators. Circulation 1996;94:2807–2816.
7. Packer M, Colucci WS, Sackner-Bernstein JD, et al. Double-blind, placebo-controlled study of effects of carvedilol in patients with moderate to severe heart failure. The PRECISE Trial. Circulation 1996;94:2793–2799.
8. CAST Investigators. Special report: effect of encainide and flecainide on mortality in a randomized trial of arrhythmia suppression after myocardial infarction. N Engl J Med 1989;321:406–412.
9. Cardiac Arrhythmia Suppression Trial II Investigators. Effect of the antiarrhythmic agent moricizine on survival after myocardial infarction. N Engl J Med 1992;327:227–233.
10. Singh SN, Fletcher RD, Fisher Gross S, et al. Amiodarone in patients with congestive heart failure and asymptomatic ventricular arrhythmia. Survival Trial of Antiarrhythmic Therapy in Congestive Heart Failure. N Engl J Med 1995; 333:77–82.

74 Background and Current Concepts

11. CIBIS Investigators and Committees. A randomized trial of beta-blockade in heart failure: the Cardiac Insufficiency Bisoprolol Study (CIBIS). Circulation 1994;90:1765–1773.
12. The CONSENSUS Trial Study Group. Effects of enalapril on mortality in severe congestive heart failure. Results of the Cooperative North Scandinavian Enalapril Survival Study (CONSENSUS). N Engl J Med 1987;316:1429–1435.
13. The Digitalis Investigation Group. The effect of digoxin on mortality and morbidity in patients with heart failure. N Engl J Med 1997;336:525–533.
14. Pitt B, Segal R, Martinez FA, et al. Randomised trial of losartan versus captopril in patients over 65 with heart failure. Lancet 1997;349:747–752.
15. Julian DG, Camm AJ, Frangin G, et al. Randomised trial of effect of amiodarone on mortality in patients with left-entricular dysfunction after recent myocardial infarction: EMIAT. European Myocardial Infarct Amiodarone Trial Investigators. Lancet 1997;349:667–674.
16. Massie BM, Berk MR, Brozena SC, et al. Can further benefit be achieved by adding flosequinan to patients with congestive heart failure who remain symptomatic on diuretic, digoxin, and an angiotensin-converting enzyme inhibitor? Results of the Flosequinan-ACE Inhibitor Trial (FACET). Circulation 1993;88:492–501.
17. Doval HC, Nul DR, Grancelli HO, et al. Randomized trial of low dose amiodarone in severe congestive heart failure. Grupo de Estudio de la Sobrevida en la Insuficiencia Cardiaca en Argentina (GESICA). Lancet 1994;344:493–498.
18. Gruppo Italiano per lo Studio della Sopravvivenza nell-Infarto Miocardico. GISSI-3: effects of lisinopril and transdermal glyceryl trinitrate singly and together on 6-week mortality and ventricular function after acute myocardial infarction. Lancet 1994;343:1115–1122.
19. International Study of Infarct Survival Research Group. Fourth international study of infarct survival: a randomized factorial trial assessing early oral captopril, oral mononitrate, and intravenous magnesium sulphate in 58,050 patients with suspected acute myocardial infarction. Lancet 1995;345:669–685.
20. Moss AJ, Hall J, Cannom DS, et al. Improved survival with an implanted defibrillator in patients with coronary disease at high risk for ventricular arrhythmia. Multicenter Automatic Defibrillator Implantation Trial Investigators. N Engl J Med 1996;335:1933–1940.
21. Waagstein F, Bristow MR, Snedberg K, et al. Beneficial effects of metoprolol in idiopathic dilated cardiomyopathy. Metoprolol in Dilated Cardiomyopathy (MDC) Trial Study Group. Lancet 1993;342:1441–1446.
22. The Multicenter Diltiazem Post Infarction Trial Research Group. The effect of diltiazem on mortality and reinfarction after myocardial infarction. N Engl J Med 1988;319:385–392.
23. Mason JW, O'Connell JB, Herskowitz A, et al. A clinical trial of immunosuppressive therapy for myocarditis. The Myocarditis Treatment Trial Investigators. N Engl J Med 1995;333:269–275.
24. The Pimobendan in Congestive Heart Failure (PICO) Investigators. Effect of pimobendan on exercise capacity in patients with heart failure: main results from the Pimobendan in Congestive Heart Failure (PICO) Trial. Heart 1996;76: 223–231.
25. Packer M, O'Connor CM, Ghali JK, et al. Effect of amlodipine on morbidity and mortality in severe chronic heart failure. Prospective Randomized Amlodipine Survival Evaluation Study Group. N Engl J Med 1996;335:1107–1114.
26. Hampton JR, van Veldhuisen DJ, Kleber FX, et al. Randomised study of the effect of ibopamine on survival in patients with advanced severe heart failure. Second Prospective Randomised Study of Ibopamine on Mortality and Efficacy (PRIME II) Investigators. Lancet 1997;349:971–977.
27. PROFILE Investigators Group. Prospective randomized flosequinan longevity evaluation [Abstract]. Circulation 1993;88(Suppl I):I-301.

28. Packer M, Carver JR, Rodeheffer RJ, et al. Effect of oral milrinone on mortality in severe chronic heart failure. The PROMISE Study Research Group. N Engl J Med 1991;325:1468–1475.
29. Uretsky BF, Young JB, Shahidi FE, et al. Randomized study assessing the effect of digoxin withdrawal in patients with mild to moderate chronic congestive heart failure: results of the PROVED trial. PROVED Investigative Group. J Am Coll Cardiol 1993;22:955–962.
30. Packer M, Gheorghiade M, Young J, et al. Withdrawal of digoxin from patients with chronic heart failure treated with angiotensin-converting enzyme inhibitors. N Engl J Med 1993;329:1–7.
31. Pfeffer MA, Braunwald E, Moye LA, et al. Effect of captopril on mortality and morbidity in patients with ventricular dysfunction after myocardial infarction. Results of the survival and ventricular enlargement trial. The SAFE Investigators. N Engl J Med 1992;327:669–677.
32. Ambrosioni E, Borghi C, Magnani B. The effect of the angiotensin-converting-enzyme inhibitor zofenopril on mortality and morbidity after anterior myocardial infarction. Survival of Myocardial Infarction Long-Term Evaluation (SMILE) Study Investigators. N Engl J Med 1995;332:80–85.
33. SOLVD Investigators. Effect of enalapril on mortality and the development of heart failure in asymptomatic patients with reduced left ventricular ejection fractions. N Engl J Med 1992;327:685–691.
34. SOLVD Investigators. Effect of enalapril on survival in patients with reduced left ventricular ejection fractions and congestive heart failure. N Engl J Med 1991;325:293–302.
35. Waldo AL, Camm AJ, deRuyter H, et al. Effect of d-sotalol on mortality in patients with left ventricular dysfunction after recent and remote myocardial infarction. The SWORD Investigators. Lancet 1996;348:7–12.
36. Kober L, Torp-Pedersen C, Carlsen JE, et al. A clinical trial of the angiotensin-converting-enzyme inhibitor trandolapril in patients with left ventricular dysfunction after myocardial infarction. Trandolapril Cardiac Evaluation (TRACE) Study Group. N Engl J Med 1995;333:1670–1676.
37. Feldman AM, Bristow MR, Parmley WW, et al. Effects of vesnarinone on morbidity and mortality in patients with heart failure. Vesnarinone Study Group. N Engl J Med 1993;329:149–155.
38. Cohn JN, Archibald DG, Ziesche S, et al. Effect of vasodilator therapy on mortality in chronic congestive heart failure: results of a Veterans Administration cooperative study (VeHEFT-I). N Engl J Med 1986;314:1547–1552.
39. Cohn JN, Johnson G, Ziesche S, et al. A comparison of enalapril with hydralazine-isosorbide dinitrate in the treatment of chronic congestive heart failure (VeHEFT-II). N Engl J Med 1991;325:303–310.
40. Boden WE, Ziesche S, Carson PE, et al. Rationale and design of the third vasodilator, heart failure trial (VeHEFT III): felodipine as adjunctive therapy to enalapril and loop diuretics with or without digoxin in chronic congestive heart failure. Am J Cardiol 1996;77:1078–1082.
41. Xamoterol in Severe Heart Failure Study Group. Xamoterol in severe heart failure. Lancet 1990;336:16–23.
42. Feldman A, Young JB, Bourge R, et al. Mechanism of increased mortality from vesnarinone in the severe heart failure trial (VesT). The VesT Investigators. J Am Coll Cardiol 1997;29(Suppl A):64A.

Chapter 6

Medical Issues in Revascularization in Heart Failure

Roger M. Mills Jr.

Chronic ischemic heart disease now accounts for approximately half of all patients with clinical heart failure. Intense basic and clinical research during the past two decades has dramatically changed both our understanding of the problem and the principles of its medical management. At the core of the issue lies an intriguing question: How does chronic atherosclerotic disease in the major epicardial conduit vessels produce the clinical picture of heart failure? In the mid-1970s the answer was that the atherosclerotic process slowly and inexorably worsened until coronary blood flow no longer satisfies myocardial oxygen needs. The ensuing infarction causes myocardial cell death, and with it comes irreversible heart failure. This answer was simple, clear-cut, and wrong.

The old paradigm failed to account for the following five observations, which grew out of the era of invasive and interventional cardiology and echocardiography:

1. When patients with acute myocardial infarction undergo urgent coronary angiography and thrombolytic therapy, the typical findings include obstructive thrombus superimposed on irregular but usually nonobstructive plaque.
2. After infarction occurs, geometric changes in the infarcted zone (expansion) and the remaining viable myocardium (remodeling) are clearly evident on serial echocardiographic imaging over time, despite no further ischemic events.
3. Brief episodes of myocardial ischemia, as documented by ambulatory electrocardiographic monitoring, may result in

    prolonged periods of contractile depression in the ischemic zone, commonly known as myocardial stunning.

4. Chronic ischemia may result in down regulation of mechanical activity (hibernation), which is reversible with mechanical revascularization and restoration of adequate blood flow.

5. Chronic hemodynamic decompensation per se may worsen subendocardial ischemia, and restoration of hemodynamic compensation may significantly improve global function.

This chapter reviews the evidence that revascularization may improve cardiac function, examines the various imaging modalities available as diagnostic tests for patients with ischemic heart failure, and looks at the clinical importance of ischemic heart failure and the results of treatment. Finally, recommendations for clinicians will be presented as an algorithm that summarizes practice guidelines.

EVIDENCE IN FAVOR OF REVASCULARIZATION IMPROVING MYOCARDIAL FUNCTION

Although the focus of this book is primarily on chronic heart failure, the evidence favoring urgent revascularization in patients with shock associated with acute myocardial infarction must not be overlooked. Extremely convincing evidence favors prompt revascularization with acute coronary occlusion and heart failure. Effective thrombolytic therapy has been associated with prompt decreases in left ventricular end-diastolic pressure (LVEDP), improvement in the ejection fraction, reduction of acute mitral regurgitation, and decreased mortality. Urgent revascularization with percutaneous transluminal coronary angiography (PTCA) produces similar favorable effects. Survival from cardiogenic shock associated with myocardial infarction is markedly enhanced with catheter-based intervention and revascularization. These recommendations are now sufficiently well accepted to be included in the current American College of Cardiology/American Heart Association Task Force practice guidelines (1).

Clinical observations from the mid 1980s of patients with chronic heart failure caused by coronary artery disease documented the concept of hibernating myocardium (Fig. 6.1). A zone of myocardium distal to a high-grade epicardial coronary stenosis may become hypokinetic or akinetic, with marked down regulation of contractile activity, while maintaining viability. With restoration of blood flow, the hibernating tissue gradually recovers significant contractile function.

Both surgical revascularization and successful PTCA have resulted in restoration of contractile function in previous ischemic tissue. In fact, effective therapy of unstable angina has also been demonstrated to improve left ventricular wall motion.

More recently, the Ambulatory Cardiac Ischemia Pilot (ACIP) study investigators noted frequent episodes of significant asymptomatic cardiac ischemia in patients with multivessel coronary disease (2). Clinical evidence indicates that such repetitive episodes of ischemia may result in reversible loss of contractile function, or stunning, associated with hemodynamic compromise (Fig. 6.2). As outlined

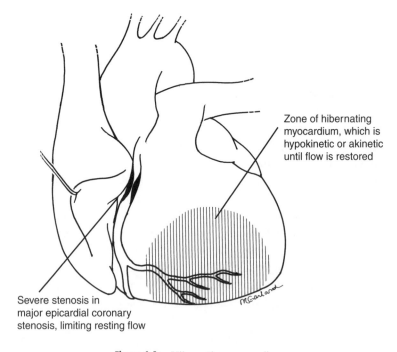

Zone of hibernating myocardium, which is hypokinetic or akinetic until flow is restored

Severe stenosis in major epicardial coronary stenosis, limiting resting flow

Figure 6.1:   Hibernating myocardium.

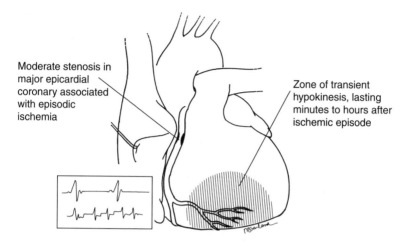

Moderate stenosis in major epicardial coronary associated with episodic ischemia

Zone of transient hypokinesis, lasting minutes to hours after ischemic episode

Figure 6.2:   Stunned myocardium.

below, the hemodynamic effects of ischemia generate a physiologic negative feedback loop, worsening the already precarious balance of coronary perfusion while increasing myocardial oxygen needs. Thus recurrent episodes of ischemia may play a role in the developing picture of ischemic cardiac failure.

DIAGNOSTIC TECHNIQUES FOR IDENTIFICATION OF VIABLE MYOCARDIUM

Once the potential for recovery of function in viable but noncontractile myocardium had been established by clinical observations, investigators turned to the problem of identifying appropriate candidates among ischemic heart failure patients for attempts at revascularization. In the nuclear medicine laboratory, this involves demonstrating a mismatch between perfusion and viability. The hallmark of hibernating myocardium in the nuclear laboratory is regional hypoperfusion with continued evidence of cellular viability.

Viability assessment requires both a blood flow study and metabolic or viability imaging. A number of techniques have evolved, including the use of thallium 201 (^{201}Tl) to generate images acquired at different times after injection, usually an early perfusion scan and a late viability scan. Alternatively, a flow imaging agent, such as

^{201}Tl or sestamibi, may be chosen for blood flow imaging and ^{18}F-fluoro-2-deoxyglucose (FDG) with high-speed single-photon emission computed tomography (SPECT) imaging used for the viability scan. If available, positron emission tomography (PET) studies may be used to generate both flow and viability scans using carbon 11 (^{11}C) acetate or FDG for metabolic imaging.

Nuclear studies require costly imaging equipment, extensive computer processing, and in the case of PET images, the ability to generate and handle short half-life radiopharmaceuticals. In addition, the studies may take several hours to several days to complete.

Unlike metabolic imaging, echocardiographic identification of myocardial viability rests on the assumption that viable but hypocontractile myocardium has contractile reserve. During positive inotropic stimulation with dobutamine, the nonfunctioning, or hypocontractile ischemic, zone will transiently improve its mechanical function. The enhanced wall motion may be detected by continuous echocardiographic imaging. In many ischemic segments, contractile reserve appears with modest inotropic stimulation. At higher levels of positive inotropic stress, mechanical dysfunction again becomes the dominant feature, owing to worsening stress-induced ischemia. This initial enhancement followed by subsequent deterioration is referred to as a biphasic response.

Technically, dobutamine stress echocardiography (DSE) offers a number of practical advantages over nuclear techniques. The entire study can be completed in a shorter time, and a complete echocardiographic examination with its wealth of structural information may be obtained at the same sitting. Drawbacks include the lack of adequate acoustic windows in some patients, difficulty imaging all myocardial segments in orthogonal views, and difficulty correlating echo findings with coronary anatomy. Transesophageal imaging can overcome many of these imaging drawbacks with only a modest increase in technical complexity.

As physicians have come to appreciate Bayes's theorem and the issues of sensitivity and specificity, most studies of diagnostic techniques now employ receiver operating characteristic (ROC) curves to compare various testing modalities. Using this approach, the differences between various nuclear strategies are relatively small, with a slight but not statistically significant trend favoring the use of ^{11}C acetate and PET for viability assessment.

The data comparing ^{201}Tl assessments to DSE viability testing, the two most commonly employed modalities, involve relatively few cases and remain controversial. The clinical gold standard for these studies is a return of mechanical function after revascularization. This standard, however, introduces its own set of variables, since revascularization must be adequate to compare nuclear techniques and DSE. At present, there are no reports of large numbers of patients who were studied by both techniques and who were subjected to revascularization with documented follow-up. From the small series in the literature, nuclear techniques appear somewhat more sensitive in identifying viability, but DSE response appears to be a better predictor of improved mechanical function after revascularization.

For the practicing clinician, given currently available data, the critical issues are (a) maintaining a high degree of awareness of potentially reversible heart failure with advanced ischemic disease and (b) consistently employing the diagnostic technology available locally to develop a good appreciation for the results in clinical practice.

CLINICAL IMPORTANCE OF MYOCARDIAL VIABILITY ASSESSMENT

Current estimates indicate that between 400,000 and 500,000 patients experience the onset of overt heart failure each year in the United States. Many of these patients are elderly, and many do not undergo complete cardiovascular diagnostic evaluation. However, based on numerous series, it appears justifiable to attribute approximately half of this disease burden to chronic ischemic heart disease.

The clinician faced with an individual patient must first ask, "Would this patient be a candidate for either catheter-based or direct surgical revascularization if suitable lesions are present?" In situations in which age or extensive comorbidity preclude any attempt at mechanical revascularization, a search for chronic ischemic disease and viability is not justified.

On the other hand, heart failure alone, even with advanced left ventricular systolic dysfunction, does not pose a contraindication to a full-diagnostic evaluation. In a series of 59 patients with advanced coronary disease referred as potential candidates for orthotopic cardiac transplantation or for heart failure care at the University of Florida, 58% had evidence of significant myocardial viability, and 29% subsequently underwent revascularization with a 30-day survival rate of 86%. Major factors limiting revascularization included lack of available bypass conduits for reoperation and extensive distal coronary disease in about 10% of cases (3).

Based on the findings in this very ill group, with an average ejection fraction of approximately 17%, as many as half of all patients with ischemic heart failure might be expected to have substantial viability, on the order of 100,000 patients per year in the United States. Because this subset with advanced disease represents approximately one-quarter of the entire population with new onset heart failure and because patients with multivessel coronary disease and impaired left ventricular systolic function have a particularly dire long-term prognosis, efforts to identify and appropriately treat these patients are important quality indicators.

A number of physiologic issues important in the long-term management of these patients frequently go unrecognized. Figure 6.3 shows the coronary perfusion gradient that normally exists across the myocardium and the effects of epicardial coronary disease, left heart failure, and a combination of both on the perfusion gradient. Elevation of LVEDP associated with heart failure significantly decreases the perfusion pressure in the myocardium served by critically stenotic vessels. In this setting, limitation of inflow by epicardial coronary disease and compromise of outflow by elevated LVEDP combine to severely compromise myocardial nutrient blood flow and myocardial function. Relief of either inflow or outflow compromise or both may substantially improve global function.

Clinically, these observations justify continued vigorous medical management for heart failure patients who undergo revascularization. The revascularization procedure alone does not usually restore ventricular function to normal, but it often offers enough improvement so that heart failure may be managed successfully with angiotensin-converting enzyme (ACE) inhibitors and modest diuresis.

CLINICAL RECOMMENDATIONS

Defining the importance of ischemic but viable myocardium in precipitating and maintaining the heart failure state requires careful

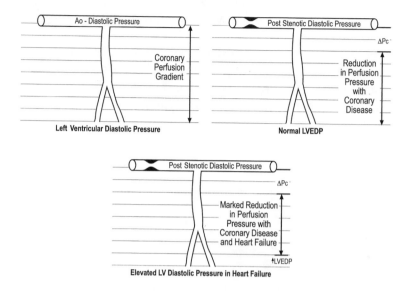

Figure 6.3: The normal coronary perfusion gradient and the effects of epicardial coronary disease, left heart failure, and a combination of both on the perfusion gradient.

clinical studies. As always, a detailed history and physical examination forms the basis for any further investigations. The primary laboratory database must include a reliable assessment of ventricular function, usually via a resting two-dimensional and Doppler echocardiographic examination; ambulatory monitoring for 24 to 48 h will often demonstrate asymptomatic ST depression or significant arrhythmia.

If clinical evidence supports a working diagnosis of ischemic heart disease with heart failure and if the individual patient is a candidate for revascularization, then a diagnostic right *and* left heart catheterization with selective coronary angiography should be performed to confirm the clinical diagnosis, assess the technical possibilities of revascularization, and document hemodynamic status. If revascularization is technically possible, then an appropriate myocardial viability investigation should follow. If the patient's echocardiographic examination is technically satisfactory, a DSE would be an appropriate study based on current evaluation. If not, transesophageal

DSE and ^{201}Tl studies are available in most hospitals throughout the United States.

For adult heart failure patients with no clear-cut working diagnosis, cardiac catheterization and coronary angiography should be considered if the individual is a potential transplant recipient or is a diabetic, who might be prone to silent coronary disease. Also con-

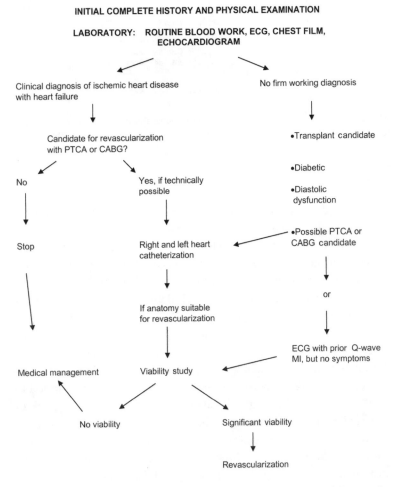

INITIAL COMPLETE HISTORY AND PHYSICAL EXAMINATION

LABORATORY: ROUTINE BLOOD WORK, ECG, CHEST FILM, ECHOCARDIOGRAM

Clinical diagnosis of ischemic heart disease with heart failure

No firm working diagnosis

Candidate for revascularization with PTCA or CABG?

•Transplant candidate

No

Yes, if technically possible

•Diabetic

•Diastolic dysfunction

Stop

Right and left heart catheterization

•Possible PTCA or CABG candidate

or

If anatomy suitable for revascularization

ECG with prior Q-wave MI, but no symptoms

Medical management

Viability study

No viability

Significant viability

Revascularization

Figure 6.4: Algorithm of practice guidelines. *CABG,* coronary artery bypass graft.

sider catheterization if clinical evaluation indicates significant diastolic dysfunction that might be attributed to repetitive stunning. In all these cases, catheterization will provide important anatomic and physiologic information for long-term management. On the other hand, if the history and routine electrocardiography indicate prior Q wave myocardial infarction, but the patient has no current ischemic symptoms, a DSE as a screening test for myocardial viability would be an appropriate first step. If left ventricular systolic function is markedly impaired with no evidence of hibernating viable myocardium, then a diagnostic coronary angiogram may not be appropriate. These recommendations are summarized in Figure 6.4.

SUMMARY

Given the enormous expense of heart failure care, the extraordinarily poor prognosis of heart failure caused by coronary disease, the relatively high incidence of myocardial viability, and the good outcomes associated with mechanical revascularization, the argument for careful investigation of patients with ischemic heart failure becomes compelling. When individual patients slip from New York Heart Association class II to III, a number of clinical responses should be triggered, including a comprehensive reassessment of the diagnostic process, a careful search for all potentially treatable causes of the patients' decompensation, and a thorough reassessment of the medical maintenance program. An understanding of the physiologic process of coronary disease and an unrelentingly vigorous diagnostic strategy are required to achieve optimal outcomes.

REFERENCES

1. American College of Cardiology/American Heart Association Task Force. Guidelines for the evaluation and management of heart failure. J Am Coll Cardiol 1995;26:1376–1398.
2. Davies RF, Goldberg AD, Forman S, et al. Asymptomatic Cardiac Ischemia Pilot (ACIP) study two-year follow-up: outcomes of patients randomized to initial strategies of medical therapy versus revascularization. Circulation 1997;95:2037–2043.
3. Mills RM Jr, Calhoun WB, Drane WE. Clinical importance of viability assessment in chronic ischemic heart failure. Clin Cardiol 1996;19:367–369.

SUGGESTED READING

Beller GA. Comparison of ^{201}Tl scintigraphy and low-dose dobutamine echocardiography for the non-invasive assessment of myocardial viability. Circulation 1996;94:2681–2684.

Bonow RO. Identification of viable myocardium. Circulation 1996;94:2674–2680.

McGhie AI, Weyman A. Searching for hibernating myocardium. Time to reevaluate investigative strategies? Circulation 1996;94:2685–2688.

Mills RM Jr, Pepine CJ. Heart failure secondary to coronary artery disease. In: Greenberg BH, Hosenpud JD, eds., Congestive heart failure. New York: Springer-Verlag, 1994:177–195.

Patel B, Kloner RA, Przyklenk K, Braunwald E. Post-ischemic myocardial "stunning." A clinically relevant phenomenon. Ann Int Med 1988;108:626–628.

Rahimtoola SH. The hibernating myocardium. Am Heart J 1989;117:211–221.

Chapter 7

Management of Atrial Fibrillation

Jamie B. Conti

EPIDEMIOLOGY OF ATRIAL FIBRILLATION

The incidence of atrial fibrillation rises sharply with age and underlying cardiovascular disease (1). Between 2 and 4% of the entire U.S. population will eventually have atrial fibrillation, including 13 to 15% of those over the age of 80. Atrial fibrillation is clearly associated with increased morbidity and mortality, owing in part to its association with increasing age, underlying heart disease, and the increased risk of thromboembolic events.

The Framingham Study provided the best data on the incidence, prevalence, and predictors of atrial fibrillation (1). During 22 years of follow-up, 2325 men and 2866 women had biennial electrocardiograms and cardiac risk factor screening. The investigators defined atrial fibrillation as chronic if it appeared on one or more consecutive electrocardiograms.

During the study, 49 men and 49 women developed chronic atrial fibrillation. The incidence of atrial fibrillation increased significantly with increasing age, and there was no difference in incidence between men and women. Atrial fibrillation developed most often in patients with previously diagnosed cardiovascular disease, specifically hypertension, congestive heart failure (CHF), rheumatic valvular disease, and coronary artery disease (CAD); although only rheumatic heart disease and congestive heart failure were powerful predictors of its occurrence. Hypertension alone was not a strong predictor; however, hypertensive heart disease with left ventricular hypertrophy was.

The Manitoba Follow-Up Study (MFUS) followed 3983 male aviation recruits beginning in 1948 and recorded the results of the subjects' routine medical examinations (2). The investigators estimated the age-specific incidence of atrial fibrillation (males only) and identified risk factors for the development of atrial fibrillation. Consistent with the Framingham data, MFUS found that the incidence of atrial fibrillation increased with age, from less than 0.5/1000 person-years before the age of 50 years to 2.3/1000 person-years by age 60 to 16.9/1000 person-years by age 85. Individuals with noted cardiac conditions, including hypertension; CAD; CHF; and less commonly, pericarditis and congenital heart disease had an increased risk of atrial fibrillation compared to those without organic heart disease.

THE PHYSIOLOGIC PROBLEMS OF ATRIAL FIBRILLATION

Although not usually acutely life threatening, atrial fibrillation is not benign. Negative physiologic effects associated with atrial fibrillation include (*a*) loss of atrial contribution to ventricular filling, (*b*) lack of rate control associated with variable diastolic filling, (*c*) lack of rate response to exercise, and (*d*) tachycardia-induced left ventricular dysfunction (LVD) (Fig. 7.1). Control of each of these physiologic issues should be part of the decision-making process when evaluating therapy for patients.

Loss of Atrial Contribution to Ventricular Filling

Sir Thomas Lewis first described the effect of atrial contraction on ventricular filling when he noted a decrease in cardiac output

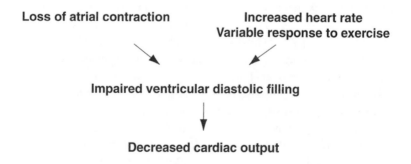

Figure 7.1: Hemodynamic consequences of atrial fibrillation.

during atrial fibrillation in dogs (3). He attributed this to an increase in heart rate; however, subsequent investigators have demonstrated that appropriately timed atrial systole makes a significant contribution to cardiac output (4). This becomes particularly important in clinical heart failure states associated with impaired diastolic filling, e.g., left ventricular hypertrophy, restrictive cardiomyopathy, and mitral stenosis.

Lack of Rate Control

In addition to the loss of the atrial contribution to ventricular filling, the characteristically irregular ventricular response to atrial fibrillation results in highly variable diastolic filling times and thus marked variations in stroke volume. Acutely, a decrease in diastolic filling time may lead to increased left atrial pressure, particularly in patients with restriction to filling from ventricular hypertrophy or coronary disease, and can precipitate myocardial ischemia or pulmonary edema (4).

With chronically rapid ventricular rates, patients may develop heart failure secondary to a tachycardia-induced cardiomyopathy. This has been well described with other supraventricular tachycardias (5) but is less frequently recognized with atrial fibrillation (6). LVD in some patients with atrial fibrillation may represent the effect of the uncontrolled ventricular response, not the cause of the arrhythmia. Since chronic uncontrolled tachycardia may result in profound left ventricular dysfunction, adequate rate control is critical. With adequate rate control, ejection fraction may improve over the following 1 to 12 months, although the damage is sometimes irreversible (5).

Rate Response to Exercise

Exercise intolerance associated with atrial fibrillation may reflect an inadequate rate response to exercise. In addition to the negative inotropic and chronotropic effects from drugs used to slow ventricular response, older patients with atrial fibrillation frequently have associated sinus and AV nodal dysfunction. Although the ventricular response to atrial fibrillation at rest may appear well controlled, the heart rate cannot increase normally with exercise. Rate response to exercise is easily assessed using electrocardiographic monitoring and exercise treadmill testing. Both are acceptable for evaluating the adequacy of rate response; electrocardiographic monitoring has the advantage of allowing the physician to assess the patient's rate response with normal activity, and formal exercise testing allows more precise quantitation of physical capacity. Patients should be counseled to continue routine activity while wearing the electrocardiographic monitor to get a valid estimate of rate response throughout the day.

CARDIOVERSION STRATEGIES

Cardioversion implies therapeutic restoration of sinus rhythm by drugs, electrical shock, or a combination of both. Before any attempt at cardioversion, the physician should ascertain the duration of atrial fibrillation and the risk of embolic stroke. Traditionally, patients who have had atrial fibrillation longer than 48 h are given anticoagulants for 3 to 4 weeks before cardioversion to decrease the risk of embolic stroke with restoration of atrial function, regardless of the method of cardioversion. Recently, transesophageal echocardiography (TEE) has provided an alternative (Fig. 7.2).

Manning et al. (7) performed TEE on 230 patients with atrial fibrillation of more than 2 days' duration. They assessed the safety of TEE for visualizing atrial thrombi before cardioversion and used the results of TEE to proceed to early cardioversion for patients without detectable atrial thrombi. With TEE, they found atrial thrombi in 34 patients. A total of 186 of 196 patients without atrial thrombi had successful cardioversion with no thromboembolic events. These patients did receive heparin before the TEE and warfarin for 1 month after cardioversion. The authors concluded that cardioversion of atrial fibrillation of unknown duration with TEE guidance, in conjunction with short-term anticoagulation, was as safe as conventional therapy and facilitated early cardioversion of hospitalized patients. This strategy minimized the total duration of anticoagulation, atrial fibrillation, and atrial mechanical dysfunction.

The options for cardioversion, whether after 3 to 4 weeks of anticoagulation or with TEE screening, include chemical cardioversion, electrical cardioversion, and intracardiac catheter techniques.

Chemical Cardioversion

Chemical cardioversion can be attempted with any of the class 1A, 1C, and III antiarrhythmic drugs. No single drug has proven superior in cardioversion or in maintenance of normal sinus rhythm.

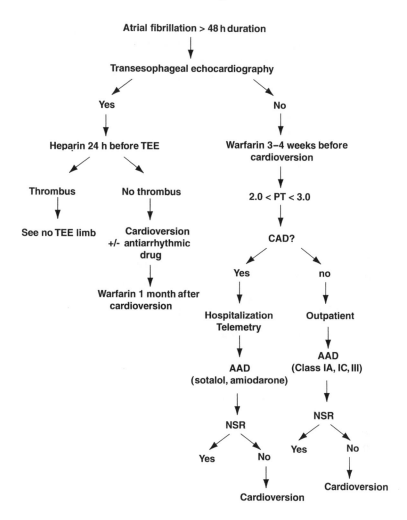

Figure 7.2: Management strategy for cardioversion of atrial fibrillation lasting more than 48 h. *PT,* prothrombin time; *AAD,* antiarrhythmic drugs; *NSR,* normal sinus rhythm.

The safety and benefits of antiarrhythmic drugs in patients with CAD and CHF have been questioned. The Cardiac Arrhythmia Suppression Trial (CAST) (8) used class 1C antiarrhythmic drugs (flecainide, encainide, and propafenone) in patients with premature ventricular contractions (PVC) after myocardial infarction. The study demonstrated a higher mortality in patients treated with drugs than in those treated with placebo. Avoidance of class 1C drugs in all patients with structural heart disease is now recommended.

A meta-analysis of a series of trials using quinidine for patients with CAD and atrial fibrillation also demonstrated higher mortality with drug therapy than with placebo (9). The Stroke Prevention in Atrial Fibrillation (SPAF) investigators demonstrated that cardiac mortality in patients with atrial fibrillation and congestive heart failure increased with antiarrhythmic drugs; in contrast, patients without heart failure tolerated class 1A drugs (quinidine, procainamide, disopyramide) 1C drugs (flecainide, encainide), and amiodarone (10).

Current data suggest that class III drugs (sotalol, amiodarone) are safest for patients with structural heart disease. The drugs have demonstrated efficacy in the treatment of atrial fibrillation, with predictable side effect profiles. Sotalol should be avoided in patients with renal failure, as it is 100% renally excreted. Hemodialysis is unpredictable and unreliable for drug removal. Because sotalol has β-blocking effects, it should be used with caution in patients with severely impaired left ventricular function or bronchospastic disease. Careful monitoring of the QT interval is essential.

When amiodarone is used for atrial fibrillation, an initial load of 600 mg daily for 1 month followed by 200 mg daily maintenance is usually effective; adverse effects may still occur at this low dose, including rare pulmonary toxicity, thyroid toxicity, liver function abnormalities, lenticular opacities, and skin discoloration. Thyroid, liver, and pulmonary function studies should be obtained every 6 months and a yearly ophthalmologic examination should be performed.

AV nodal blocking agents, such as digoxin, diltiazem, verapamil, and β-blockers, slow the ventricular response to atrial fibrillation, but do not result in conversion to sinus rhythm. Although useful in the acute management of atrial fibrillation to slow the ventricular rate and stabilize hemodynamics, AV nodal blockers are not essential to a cardioversion strategy.

Hospitalization for initiation of drug therapy depends on the underlying cardiac disease. Patients with CHF or significant CAD are at risk for developing proarrhythmic effects and require hospitalization and monitoring.

Electrical Cardioversion

Antiarrhythmic medications administered to achieve therapeutic drug levels facilitate electrical cardioversion. Elective electrical cardioversion for atrial fibrillation requires short-acting general anesthesia, with emergency resuscitation equipment easily available. For synchronized dc cardioversion, an initial energy setting of 200 J is recommended, followed by 300 and then 360 J, if needed. There is no value to repeated shocks at the same energy, and the likelihood of causing serious chest burns increases. Proper electrocardiographic synchronization should be confirmed before each attempt. Patients should be informed that risks associated with electrical cardioversion include chest wall burns, thromboembolic events, refractory arrhythmias, and the risk associated with general anesthesia.

Other Nonpharmacologic Therapy

If synchronized dc cardioversion up to 360 J for a patient on appropriate drug therapy fails to convert the patient to normal sinus rhythm, three therapeutic options remain. First, the patient can remain in chronic atrial fibrillation, managed as discussed later. A second alternative is a relatively new procedure: intracardiac defibrillation (11). This involves placing a catheter in the right atrium and delivering electrical energy directly to the atrial myocardium. The procedure has demonstrated benefit in patients with particularly wide chest cavities and increased thoracic impedance, in whom external cardioversion has failed. Risks include delivery of current directly to the atrial wall, resulting in atrial perforation with tamponade, and inadvertent ablation of the AV node.

Third, several surgical approaches now exist for treatment of atrial fibrillation; the most common and widely accepted is the maze procedure (12). The maze procedure requires multiple incisions in the atrium to electrically isolate a path from the sinus node to the atrioventricular node from atrial re-entrant circuits. Although moderately successful, this technique is not widely accepted as first-line therapy. Postoperative complications can be significant, including recurrent atrial arrhythmias in 50% of patients, fluid retention, and pericarditis. Long-term documentation of success is lacking, and a substantial number of patients undergoing this procedure require permanent pacemaker implantation. Note that postsurgical return of atrial contraction has been documented by TEE (13). Recently, the same result has been accomplished using radiofrequency catheter-based techniques; this approach is still under investigation.

MANAGEMENT OF CHRONIC ATRIAL FIBRILLATION

If cardioversion fails, or atrial fibrillation returns, the patient is faced with remaining in chronic atrial fibrillation or continuing to have troublesome episodes of paroxysmal atrial fibrillation. Management of these patients can be difficult, but there are still several therapeutic strategies from which to choose (Fig. 7.3).

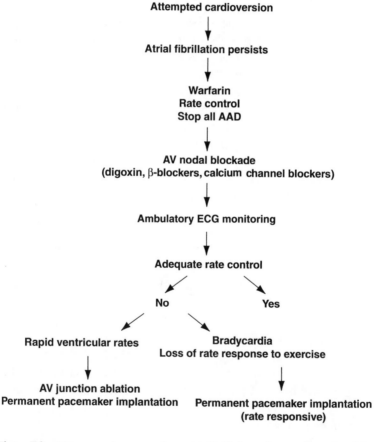

Figure 7.3: Management strategy for atrial fibrillation when cardioversion fails. *AAD,* antiarrhythmic drugs.

Medical Therapy

Continued medical therapy is an option. Although antiarrhythmic drugs have failed, AV nodal blockade to control ventricular response is still important. Useful drugs in this situation include β-blockers, calcium channel blockers, and digoxin. If the patient has coexisting LVD and atrial fibrillation, digoxin is a good first choice and may provide adequate rate control at rest. However, digoxin provides little rate control during exercise, and addition of β-blockers or calcium channel blockers is usually necessary. These may not be well tolerated in patients with significant LVD.

If medical management is pursued, documentation of rate control during exercise should be obtained with a 24-h electrocardiographic monitor or exercise testing. Note that if a patient has failed an antiarrhythmic medication and will remain in atrial fibrillation, antiarrhythmic drugs given for maintenance of sinus rhythm or prophylaxis against atrial fibrillation should be discontinued. In particular, amiodarone and sotalol should not be used solely for rate control.

Pacing

Achieving adequate AV nodal blockade with reasonable doses of oral AV nodal blocking agents is not always easy or even possible. Because all AV nodal blockers are negative inotropic agents, they may exacerbate CHF at effective doses. In addition, many patients with atrial fibrillation have associated sinus and AV nodal dysfunction and require permanent pacing to provide a stable resting heart rate and appropriate rate response with activity.

The optimal pacing mode for patients with atrial fibrillation is a topic of considerable interest. Prospective randomized trials are still ongoing, but observational evidence suggests that DDD pacing (rather than the VVI mode) may prevent recurrence of atrial fibrillation in patients predisposed to this arrhythmia. Investigators speculate that atrial pacing helps maintain a high degree of exit block from all subsidiary atrial pacemakers and thereby reduces atrial ectopy; definitive data to support this hypothesis are lacking (14). There is no evidence that VVI pacing per se causes atrial fibrillation.

Pacing and Ablation

In selected cases, radiofrequency catheter AV junction ablation or modification combined with permanent rate-responsive ventricular pacemaker implantation provides definitive therapy for patients with chronic atrial fibrillation, allowing absolute rate control and the ability to prevent bradycardia (15). When control of the ventricular rate remains inadequate despite several AV nodal blockers or when AV nodal blockers are poorly tolerated, AV junction ablation with permanent pacemaker implantation offers a particularly attractive alternative, because it provides good rate control without medication. Antiarrhythmic drugs, which can contribute significantly to patients' CHF symptoms because of their negative inotropic properties, can also be discontinued.

Patients with chronic atrial fibrillation are paced with a single ventricular lead, and their pacer is programmed in the VVIR mode; whereas those with paroxysmal atrial fibrillation are paced with an atrial and a ventricular lead, with the generator in the DDDR mode. Mode switching capabilities should be available to prevent tracking of rapid atrial fibrillation. Both physician and patient should carefully consider the decision between drug therapy and permanent ablative therapy. AV junction ablation is not completely benign; sudden cardiac death may complicate this procedure. In addition, patients must accept permanent pacemaker dependence. Factors influencing the decision include previous adverse experiences with drug therapy, proarrhythmic effects of antiarrhythmic medications, exacerbation of CHF by negative inotropic drugs, symptoms (frequency of hospitalization and poor exercise tolerance), and the desire to be free of drug therapy.

ANTICOAGULATION

Epidemiologic Link between Atrial Fibrillation and Embolic Stroke

The Framingham Study examined the impact of nonrheumatic atrial fibrillation, hypertension, CAD, and CHF on the incidence of stroke in 5070 patients (16). Follow-up was 34 years, during which time patients were examined every 2 years. The purpose of the investigation was to assess whether atrial fibrillation was truly a risk marker for stroke. No attempt was made to distinguish between thrombotic and embolic strokes.

These investigators found that nonrheumatic atrial fibrillation carried a significantly increased risk of ischemic stroke. In the presence of CAD, the incidence of stroke was more than doubled; in the presence of heart failure, incidence increased more than fourfold; and in the presence of atrial fibrillation, incidence increased fivefold. Of note, in patients 80 to 89 years old, the only significant predictor of stroke was atrial fibrillation.

The association of lone atrial fibrillation with stroke is controversial. *Lone atrial fibrillation* connotes atrial fibrillation in a structurally normal heart, with no precipitating events. Although the Framingham Study investigators found that nonrheumatic atrial fibrillation was associated with significantly increased mortality (greater than 5 times that of the general population), the atrial fibrillation patients also had CHF and CAD. In a subsequent report, the investigators found a fourfold higher rate of stroke in patients with isolated atrial fibrillation, but 32% of the patients had pre-existing hypertension, a well-established risk factor for stroke.

In contrast, Kopecky et al. (17) studied 97 patients with lone atrial fibrillation in a cohort of 3623 patients with atrial fibrillation. Of the lone fibrillators, 21% had an isolated episode of atrial fibrillation, 58% had paroxysmal atrial fibrillation, and 22% had chronic atrial fibrillation. These investigators found a low incidence of stroke in the lone fibrillators and no difference in stroke rate with recurrent paroxysms versus chronic atrial fibrillation. They concluded that patients under the age of 60 with lone atrial fibrillation had a low risk of stroke and that routine anticoagulation may not be warranted for this small group.

Most recently, the SPAF investigators reported on 568 patients randomized to placebo treatment in the SPAF I study (18). Patients under 60 years of age without clinical risk factors (hypertension, CHF, or previous thromboembolism) were at low risk for stroke. The investigators concluded that the dangers of anticoagulation with warfarin may outweigh the benefits for this subgroup of low-risk patients.

Given all available data, atrial fibrillation in the presence of related risk factors is associated with stroke. Clear-cut benefits of warfarin therapy for the prevention of stroke have been demonstrated in atrial fibrillation patients over the age of 60 and in those under the age of 60 with associated hypertension, diabetes, CHF, or previous stroke (Fig. 7.4).

Anticoagulation Trials

Over the past 5 years, several randomized multicenter trials have helped to clarify important clinical issues regarding antithrombotic therapy for stroke prevention in patients with atrial fibrillation. This section specifically discusses the SPAF I, II, and III studies (18–20); the Copenhagen Atrial Fibrillation, Aspirin, Anticoagulation study (AFASAK) (21), and the European Atrial Fibrillation Trial (EAFT) (22).

SPAF I

SPAF I, a multicenter randomized trial, compared 325 mg/day aspirin (double-blind) or adjusted-dose warfarin with placebo for prevention of ischemic stroke and systemic embolism in 1330 patients with either chronic or paroxysmal atrial fibrillation. The warfarin dose was adjusted to prolong the patients' prothrombin time (PT) to between 1.3 and 1.8 that of control (international normalized ratio, INR = 2.0–4.5). The study demonstrated that both aspirin

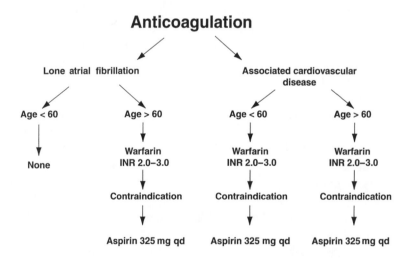

Figure 7.4: Anticoagulation recommendations for patients with and without risk factors for stroke.

and warfarin were effective in reducing ischemic stroke risk in patients with atrial fibrillation and that the risk of bleeding was not significantly different among the aspirin, warfarin, and placebo groups. Subgroup analysis suggested that aspirin was not effective for patients older than 75 years of age.

SPAF II

The SPAF II trial followed the patients who had been randomized in SPAF I to either aspirin or warfarin therapy and randomized the patients who originally had been assigned to placebo to receive either aspirin or warfarin. An additional 419 patients were recruited. The SPAF II investigators concluded that warfarin was more effective than aspirin for stroke prevention; however, the warfarin-treated group also had a higher rate of intracranial hemorrhage, particularly in patients over 75 years of age.

SPAF III

SPAF III study compared low-dose warfarin (INR = 1.3 to 1.5) plus aspirin (325 mg) to standard warfarin therapy (INR = 2.0 to 3.0) for prevention of thromboembolic events. The report indicated that standard warafin therapy was approximately 3 times more effective in preventing thromboembolic events than was the low-dose regimen. Low-dose warfarin and aspirin therapy are not recommended for patients with atrial fibrillation.

AFASAK

AFASAK included 1007 patients with chronic nonrheumatic atrial fibrillation who were randomized to therapy with either warfarin, aspirin (75 mg), or placebo for 2 years, with thromboembolic events as a primary end point. The investigators concluded that the incidence of thromboembolic complications was significantly lower in the warfarin group compared to the aspirin and placebo groups and that anticoagulation with warfarin should be offered for stroke prophylaxis to patients with chronic nonrheumatic atrial fibrillation.

EAFT

Before the publication of the EAFT results, several other trials had demonstrated the efficacy of anticoagulation in preventing thromboembolic events in nonrheumatic atrial fibrillation. EAFT attempted to define the benefit of anticoagulation drugs or aspirin in patients with a recent transient ischemic attack or minor ischemic stroke. The investigators found that warfarin reduced the risk of recurrent thromboembolic events in patients with nonrheumatic paroxysmal or chronic atrial fibrillation more effectively than did aspirin. Aspirin was superior to placebo in those who could not tolerate warfarin.

From these studies, it seems reasonable to prescribe anticoagulants to patients with atrial fibrillation who are at moderate to high risk for stroke. Patients under the age of 60 with truly lone atrial fibrillation should not receive warfarin, as the benefit of anticoagulation is not greater than the risk of hemorrhage.

Agents: Aspirin Versus Warafin

When considering the risk of embolic stroke, there is no difference between patients with paroxysmal atrial fibrillation and chronic atrial fibrillation. In general, it is believed that patients with lone atrial fibrillation under the age of 60 may be treated with aspirin alone. However, patients under 60 years with risk factors for embolic stroke—specifically, hypertension, previous embolic stroke, LVD, and female gender—require anticoagulation with warfarin. The INR should be maintained between 2.0 and 3.0. No benefit has been demonstrated with combined aspirin and low-dose warfarin (INR = 1.2 to 1.3) (20).

Patients over age 60 with atrial fibrillation should be carefully given anticoagulants with warfarin to an INR between 2.0 and 3.0. Risk for hemorrhagic stroke increases with an INR greater than 3.0.

The best timing of anticoagulation and cardioversion is incompletely understood, although there are some generally accepted guidelines. Patients who have had atrial fibrillation for more than 48 h should receive warfarin (therapeutic levels) for 3 to 4 weeks before attempting cardioversion. Alternatively, if transesophageal echocardiography demonstrates no intracardiac thrombus, patients may undergo elective cardioversion with subsequent oral anticoagulation for 3 to 4 weeks. However, if thrombus is seen, anticoagulation for 3 to 4 weeks before cardioversion is mandatory.

Although clinically accepted as safe, little data support the practice of electively cardioverting patients without anticoagulation if the duration of the arrhythmia has been less than 48 h. In these patients, it is prudent to administer heparin as soon as atrial fibrillation is recognized and to prescribe the anticoagulate warfarin for 3 to 4 weeks after successful cardioversion.

SUMMARY

Atrial fibrillation is unquestionably associated with an increased risk of embolic stroke and with increased mortality. With increasing age and organic heart disease, the incidence of atrial fibrillation increases. Management strategies must address three important problems associated with this arrhythmia. First, patients who experience palpitations, shortness of breath with exertion, or fatigue owing to their arrhythmia should be considered for cardioversion, either chemical or electrical. This population will benefit most from return of AV synchrony and maintenance of sinus rhythm. Their symptoms may stem from the irregularity of the rhythm (variable diastolic filling), the rate of their tachycardia, or the loss of atrial contribution to diastolic filling. In addition, patients with persistently rapid ventricular response to atrial fibrillation may be at risk for tachycardia-induced cardiomyopathy.

Second, adequate rate control is absolutely necessary for successful management of patients with chronic atrial fibrillation. Although historically atrial fibrillation was believed to result from organic heart disease, we are now increasingly aware that, in some cases, atrial fibrillation may actually cause or contribute to left ventricular dysfunction.

Finally, although many patients with atrial fibrillation are nearly asymptomatic, they still require therapy to prevent stroke. This goal is achieved most effectively with warfarin, with the exception of patients with lone atrial fibrillation. Stroke prophylaxis with warfarin is recommended for patients with organic heart disease and either chronic or paroxysmal atrial fibrillation.

Although atrial fibrillation is common, therapy is not always straightforward. Innovations in management include the maze procedure, intracardiac defibrillation, and AV node ablation with permanent pacemaker implantation. On the horizon may be catheter ablation techniques that simulate the maze procedure; they are under investigation and have shown promising initial results.

REFERENCES

1. Kannel WB, Abbott RD, Savage DD, McNamara PM. Epidemiologic features of chronic atrial fibrillation: the Framingham Study. N Engl J Med 1982;306:1018–1022.
2. Krahn AD, Manfreda J, Tate RB, Mathewson FAL. The natural history of atrial fibrillation: incidence, risk factors, and prognosis in the Manitoba Follow-Up Study. Am J Med 1995;98:476–484.
3. Lewis T. Fibrillation of the auricles; its effects upon the circulation. J Exp Med 1912;16:395.
4. Naito M, David D, Michelson EL, et al. The hemodynamic consequences of cardiac arrhythmias: evaluation of the relative roles of abnormal atrioventricular sequencing, irregularity of ventricular rhythm and atrial fibrillation in a canine model. Am Heart J 1983;106:284–291.
5. Packer DL, Bardy GH, Worley SJ, et al. Tachycardia-induced cardiomyopathy: a reversible form of left ventricular dysfunction. Am J Cardiol 1986;57:563–570.
6. Grogan M, Smith HC, Gersh BJ, Wood DL. Left ventricular dysfunction due to atrial fibrillation in patients initially believed to have idiopathic dilated cardiomyopathy. Am J Cardiol 1992;69:1570–1573.
7. Manning WJ, Silverman DI, Keighley CS, et al. Transesophageal echocardiographically facilitated early cardioversion from atrial fibrillation using short-term anticoagulation: final results of a prospective 4.5-year study. J Am Coll Cardiol 1995;25:1354–1361.
8. Echt DS, Liebson PR, Mitchell LB, et al. Mortality and morbidity in patients receiving encainide, flecainide or placebo. The Cardiac Arrhythmia Suppression Trial. N Engl J Med 1991;324:781–788.
9. Coplen SE, Antmann EM, Berlin JA, et al. Efficacy and safety of quinidine therapy for maintenance of sinus rhythm after cardioversion: a meta-analysis of randomized controlled trials. Circulation 1990;82:1106–1116.
10. Flaker GC, Blackshear JL, McBride R, et al. Anthiarrhythmic drug therapy and cardia mortality in atrial fibrillation. The Stroke Prevention in Atrial Fibrillation Investigators. J Am Coll Cardiol 1992;20:527–532.
11. Levy, S, Lauribe P, Dolla E, et al. A randomized comparison of external and internal cardioversion of chronic atrial fibrillation. Circulation 1992;86:1415–1420.
12. Cox JL. The surgical treatment of atrial fibrillation J Thorac Cardiovasc Surg 1991;101:584–592.
13. Cox JL, Boineau JP, Schuessler RB, et al. Five-year experience with the maze procedure for atrial fibrillation. J Thorac Cardiovasc Surg 1993;56:814–823.
14. Sgarbossa EB, Pinski SL, Maloney JD, et al. Chronic atrial fibrillation and stroke in paced patients with sick sinus syndrome. Relevance of clinical characteristics and pacing modalities. Circulation 1993;88:1045–1053.
15. Langberg JJ, Chin MC, Rosenqvist M, et al. Catheter ablation of the atrioventricular junction with radiofrequency energy. Circulation 1989;80:1527–1535.
16. Wolf PA, Abbott RD, Kannel WB. Atrial fibrillation as an independent risk factor for stroke: the Framingham Study. Stroke 1991;22:983–988.
17. Kopecky SL, Gersh BJ, Phil D, et al. The natural history of lone atrial fibrillation. A population-based study over three decades. N Engl J Med 1987;317:669–674.
18. Stroke Prevention in Atrial Fibrillation Investigators. Stroke Prevention in Atrial Fibrillation Study: final results. Circulation 1991;84:527–539.
19. Stroke Prevention in Atrial Fibrillation Investigators. Warfarin versus aspirin for prevention of thromboembolism in atrial fibrillation: Stroke Prevention in Atrial Fibrillation II Study. Lancet 1994;343:687–691.
20. Cowburn P, Cleland JG. SPAF-III results. Eur Heart J 1996;17:1129.
21. Petersen P, Boysen G, Godtfredsen J, et al. Placebo-controlled randomised trial of warfarin and aspirin for prevention of thromboembolic complications in chronic

atrial fibrillation. The Copenhagen AFASAK Study. Lancet 1989;1(8631):175–178.

22. The European Atrial Fibrillation Trial Study Group. Optimal oral anticoagulant therapy in patients with nonrheumatic atrial fibrillation and recent cerebral ischemia. N Engl J Med 1995;333:5–10.

SUGGESTED READING

Middlekauff HR, Stevenson WG, Stevenson LW. Prognostic significance of atrial fibrillation in advanced heart failure: A study of 390 patients. Circulation 1991; 84:40–48.

Prystowsky EN, Benson DW, Fuster V, et al. Management of patients with atrial fibrillation. A statement for healthcare professionals from the subcommittee on electrocardiography and electrophysiology, American Heart Association. Circulation 1996;93:1262–1277.

Chapter 8

Management of the Patient at Risk for Sudden Cardiac Death

Anne B. Curtis

Sudden cardiac syndrome may account for as much as half of the total cause-specific mortality in patients with heart failure. In most cases, ventricular fibrillation of patients with chronic heart failure precipitates sudden death. Rapid sustained ventricular tachycardia produces only a small minority of cardiac arrests; however, a few beats of ventricular tachycardia often precede ventricular fibrillation. Occasionally, asystole or profound bradycardia has been documented at the time of demise. This is more likely to occur in a patient with end-stage congestive heart failure.

Overall, atherosclerotic coronary artery disease (CAD) is responsible for 80% of all sudden cardiac deaths. Less common causes include hypertrophic cardiomyopathy, valvular heart disease, inflammatory and infiltrative cardiomyopathies, congenital heart disease, and idiopathic cardiomyopathy. Sudden cardiac death (SCD) may occur with characteristic electrocardiographic findings, such as AV block and the prolonged QT syndromes. In heart failure patients, prolonged QT syndrome is usually acquired, caused by drugs or electrolyte abnormalities. Other uncommon causes of cardiac arrest, such as ventricular pre-excitation and coronary artery anomalies, are most often found in patients without structural heart disease and are not typically concerns in patients with chronic heart failure.

The overwhelming majority of patients do not survive a cardiac arrest. After successful resuscitation, however, the risk of recurrent sudden death within 1 year is approximately 30%. To significantly improve survival in patients with serious ventricular dysfunction, we must appropriately evaluate and treat patients who have survived an episode of cardiac arrest. In addition, the much larger population of patients at risk for SCD who have not yet had overt arrhythmias must be identified and an optimal treatment program initiated.

DIAGNOSTIC TECHNIQUES

A variety of invasive and noninvasive tests help with risk stratification in patients with heart disease, evaluation of arrhythmic substrates in patients who have had life-threatening arrhythmias, and with guiding therapy.

Noninvasive Techniques

Electrocardiographic Monitoring

The technique of ambulatory continuous electrocardiographic monitoring involves continuously recording all cardiac electrical activity for a finite period, usually 24 h, and reviewing arrhythmias and symptoms during that time. The advantage of the technique lies in the ability to quantitate all arrhythmias during the recording period. The disadvantage is that it is helpful only when arrhythmias occur during the recording period. When patients have infrequent symptoms, event monitors may prove more useful.

Indications for electrocardiographic monitoring for ventricular arrhythmias include evaluation of symptoms and evaluation of therapy. A patient may complain of symptoms, such as palpitations or dizziness, for which electrocardiographic correlation is desired. Documentation of the cause of a complaint is a requisite for appropriate treatment. Alternatively, a patient may have known arrhythmias, and quantitation of frequency and characterization of the type of arrhythmia are desired either as baseline information or to determine the efficacy of therapy.

Event recorders are useful for documenting the cardiac rhythm during transient symptoms such as dizziness. Two types of event recorders are commonly available. The postevent recorder, which is the more familiar, is either placed over the chest or connected by wrist electrodes when symptoms occur. It is useful for patients whose symptoms last long enough for placement of the recorder (Fig. 8.1). In addition, the patient must not have symptoms, i.e., syncope, that preclude placement of the monitor.

For severe symptoms or very short-lived symptoms, the loop recorder is a better choice. With this technique, the event recorder

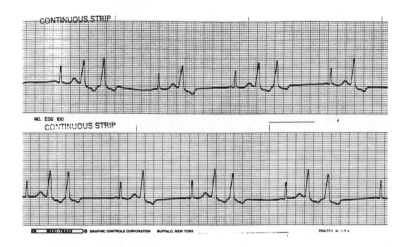

Figure 8.1: Event monitor recording from a patient with a nonischemic cardiomyopathy and complaints of dizziness. Although he had experienced premature ventricular contractions (PVCs), it was unclear if they were actually responsible for his symptoms. During an episode of dizziness outside the hospital, the patient transmitted a recording showing a trigeminal pattern, with two PVCs for every sinus beat. His effective sinus rate was extremely bradycardic. Amiodarone therapy was initiated; within 3 weeks the patient had no more than two PVCs/min, his sinus rate had increased to 60 beats/min, and the dizziness had resolved.

is attached to the patient at all times, much like a continuous electrocardiographic monitor. The cardiac rhythm is continually recorded and an ECG loop is updated. At the time symptoms occur, activating the device freezes the recording for a programmable period of time before and after activation. The ability to retain information up to 1 min *before* the button was pressed is ideal for patients with transient but hemodynamically significant arrhythmias. Both types of event recorders transmit over a telephone line to a monitoring service for electrocardiographic interpretation and notification of the physician.

Signal-Averaged Electrocardiography

Signal-averaged electrocardiography detects late potentials and low amplitude signals at the terminal portion of the QRS complex that are often present in patients with serious ventricular arrhythmias. The technique uses orthogonal XYZ leads to acquire 100 to 200 QRS complexes, which are then amplified, filtered, and digitized.

The digitized signals are aligned and summed to yield the composite signal-averaged ECG. The signal-averaging process rejects electrical artifact or noise, which otherwise obscures the late potentials. Examples of normal and abnormal signal-averaged ECGs are shown in Figure 8.2.

Patients who have had sustained ventricular tachycardia or fibrillation frequently have abnormal signal-averaged ECGs. Although most patients who have had a sustained arrhythmia certainly do not need a signal-averaged ECG for risk stratification, a signal-averaged ECG may be useful in selected cases. For example, when a patient has suffered a life-threatening ventricular arrhythmia while taking an antiarrhythmic drug, the question of proarrhythmia from the drug often arises. In other words, Has the antiarrhythmic drug aggravated an arrhythmia rather than suppressing it? Since antiarrhythmic drugs do not alter late potentials, an abnormal signal-averaged ECG might provide evidence that the patient has an underlying substrate for an arrhythmia and that discontinuation of the antiarrhythmic drug may not be sufficient to protect the patient (1).

The signal-averaged ECG is most commonly used for risk stratification. After myocardial infarction, a normal signal-averaged ECG is associated with an extremely low risk for arrhythmic events. An abnormal signal-averaged ECG increases the likelihood that a patient will have a serious arrhythmia in follow-up. In one study, the risk of a serious arrhythmia was as high as 50% if the patient also had reduced systolic function and ventricular arrhythmias on continuous electrocardiographic monitoring (2).

In a patient with structural heart disease and unexplained syncope, an abnormal signal-averaged ECG increases the likelihood that the patient will have inducible ventricular tachycardia at electrophysiologic study. With bundle branch block, late potentials may be masked, and there is a lack of general agreement on criteria for interpretation of the signal-averaged ECG. Frequency domain analysis may prove useful in such patients in the future.

Heart Rate Variability

The sinus rate in humans reflects changes in autonomic input to the sinus node. Heart rate variability may be quantified by recording all RR intervals over a period of time, usually a day, and converting the intervals to a "power spectrum" by Fourier transformation. The

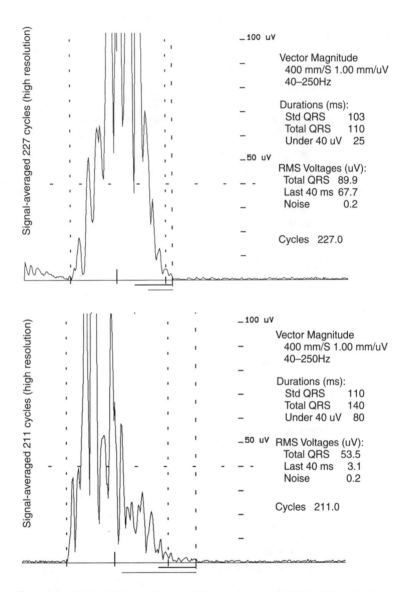

Figure 8.2: Normal (**A**) and abnormal (**B**) signal-averaged ECGs. When the filter settings are 40 to 250 Hz, a signal-averaged ECG is normal if the total QRS duration is less than 115 ms, the duration of the low amplitude signal (LAS) is less than 38 ms, and the root mean square (RMS) voltage of the terminal 40 ms is greater than 20 μV.

different frequency components of the power spectrum may then be analyzed.

Vagal tone, an important component of autonomic input to the heart, protects the heart by reducing the incidence of ventricular arrhythmias associated with myocardial infarction. A reduction in vagal tone can be detected as reduced heart rate variability. In patients with heart failure, reduced heart rate variability is a strong predictor of mortality.

Exercise Tolerance Testing

Exercise tolerance testing has an important role in the detection of ischemia in patients with ventricular arrhythmias. Most patients with nonsustained ventricular arrhythmias should undergo a screening exercise treadmill test, or another provocative test for ischemia if a treadmill is not appropriate. (In contrast, after aborted sudden death, patients usually undergo cardiac catheterization to assess the presence and severity of CAD.)

Exercise tolerance testing is occasionally useful for patients with exercise-induced arrhythmias. Determining whether an arrhythmia is suppressed or aggravated by exercise may be important in guiding therapy and in advising a patient on activity.

Echocardiography

Echocardiography is useful for evaluation of ventricular size and function and valvular heart disease in patients with ventricular arrhythmias, whether symptomatic or not. Right ventricular dysplasia, an uncommon problem associated with life-threatening ventricular arrhythmias, may also be detected by echocardiography.

Invasive Techniques

Cardiac Catheterization

Patients with asymptomatic or mildly symptomatic ventricular arrhythmias, do not require cardiac catheterization unless noninvasive studies suggest significant structural heart disease. Catheterization data are invaluable to determine the cause of a cardiomyopathy, whether ischemic or nonischemic; the significance of valvular lesions; and the patient's hemodynamic status by intracardiac pressures.

Electrophysiologic Studies

Electrophysiologic studies involve the placement of electrode catheters in the heart for recording intracardiac electrical activity and pacing the heart. An electrophysiologic study for ventricular arrhythmias uses pacing techniques to provoke sustained ventricular arrhythmia for diagnosis and to guide treatment. The usual end point for a positive study is sustained monomorphic ventricular tachycardia (Fig. 8.3). Only in rare instances, typically when a patient has presented with a cardiac arrest, should provocation of ventricular fibrillation be considered a specific finding. In most instances, ventricular fibrillation is a nonspecific outcome of electrophysiologic study and is not used to guide therapy. Indications for electrophysiologic studies for ventricular arrhythmias are shown in Table 8.1.

There are a number of goals in an electrophysiologic study for ventricular arrhythmias: (*a*) Inducibility of the arrhythmia is deter-

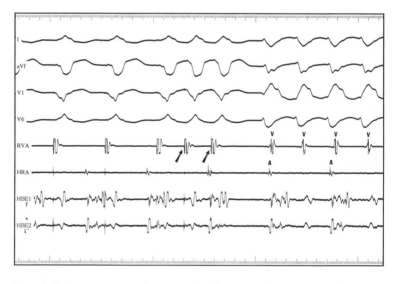

Figure 8.3: Induction of sustained monomorphic ventricular tachycardia at electrophysiologic study. **Top to bottom:** ECG leads I, aVF, V_1, and V_6, and intracardiac tracings from the right ventricular apex (RVA), high right atrium (HRA), and distal and proximal His bundle (HBE1,2). At the end of a pacing train at 120 beats/min (500 ms cycle length), two premature ventricular extrastimuli are delivered (*arrows*), with induction of sustained ventricular tachycardia. AV dissociation is evident in the recording. *A,* atrial; *V,* ventricular.

Table 8.1.   Indications for Electrophysiologic Studies for Ventricular Arrhythmias

Diagnosis
- Sustained ventricular tachycardia
- Cardiac arrest
- Wide complex tachycardia of uncertain cause
- Syncope with structural heart disease
- Nonsustained ventricular tachycardia and CAD (possibly)

Therapy
- Assessment of antiarrhythmic drug efficacy
- Evaluation of antitachycardia pacing
- Mapping to locate origin of ventricular tachycardia for catheter or surgical ablation

mined. (*b*) The diagnosis of ventricular tachycardia is confirmed by analysis of the intracardiac signals. (*c*) The feasibility of antitachycardia pacing can be assessed. Successful antitachycardia pacing may indicate that implantation of a cardioverter–defibrillator with antitachycardia pacing will be a useful therapeutic option for the patient. (*d*) Electrophysiologic studies repeated on antiarrhythmic drug therapy can prospectively assess the efficacy of the drug.

Electrophysiologic studies are not the only way to assess the efficacy of antiarrhythmic drugs. The Electrophysiologic Study Versus Electrocardiographic Monitoring Trial (ESVEM) evaluated electrophysiologic study and electrocardiographic monitoring for determining the efficacy of antiarrhythmic drugs, with arrhythmia recurrence as the end point (3). The techniques appeared equivalent. Many clinicians have used electrocardiographic monitoring to guide antiarrhythmic therapy in patients with sustained ventricular tachycardia who have frequent arrhythmias on monitoring. In this setting, the goal of antiarrhythmic therapy is to suppress at least 70% of premature ventricular contractions (PVCs) and all ventricular tachycardias. Overall, noninvasive monitoring is more commonly used to guide antiarrhythmic therapy in patients with symptomatic nonsustained arrhythmias.

TREATMENT FOR VENTRICULAR ARRHYTHMIAS

In patients with congestive heart failure and life-threatening ventricular arrhythmias, the two major therapeutic options are treatment with antiarrhythmic drugs, primarily amiodarone, and implantation of cardioverter–defibrillators.

Antiarrhythmic Drugs

There are a number of antiarrhythmic drugs available for the treatment of ventricular arrhythmias. The drugs that have activity against ventricular arrhythmias have been broadly classified into the Vaughan Williams class I and class III antiarrhythmic drugs.

The class I antiarrhythmic drugs, primarily sodium channel blockers, are further subclassified according to their effects on the electrocardiogram. The class IA antiarrhythmic drugs are quinidine, procainamide, and disopyramide. These drugs may prolong the QT interval and may cause torsades de pointes, a polymorphous ventricular tachycardia. The class IB antiarrhythmic drugs have little effect on the ECG. The two commonly used drugs in this class are lidocaine and mexiletine. The class IC antiarrhythmic drugs are flecainide and propafenone. They prolong QRS duration but have little effect on the QT interval. Neither of the IC drugs should be used in patients with significant ventricular dysfunction. Both are negative inotropic agents and carry a significant risk of proarrhythmia, manifested as monomorphic ventricular tachycardia, in patients with poor left ventricle systolic function.

The class III antiarrhythmic drugs, primarily potassium channel blockers, include bretylium, sotalol, and amiodarone. Bretylium is available only for parenteral therapy and is used only for the acute management of life-threatening ventricular arrhythmias.

Sotalol, a relatively new antiarrhythmic drug, is effective for ventricular arrhythmias (4). In the ESVEM trial, sotalol was the most effective of the antiarrhythmic drugs tested, yielding the lowest recurrence rate for ventricular tachycardia (5). Sotalol, along with amiodarone, has become one of the most frequently used drugs for the treatment of ventricular arrhythmias. The drug is a negative inotropic agent, partly owing to its β-blocking activity, and must be used cautiously in patients with reduced ventricular function.

Amiodarone is now available both orally and parenterally. The intravenous form is used for the acute management of patients with ventricular arrhythmias, most typically in patients with frequently recurring life-threatening ventricular arrhythmias or those who cannot take the drug orally (6). The expensive intravenous drug does not yield therapeutic blood levels faster than the oral formulation and offers no real advantage in most patients. Amiodarone is effective for both supraventricular and ventricular arrhythmias, although it has FDA approval only for the latter. It is probably the single most useful antiarrhythmic drug in patients with significant ventricular dysfunction. Its efficacy for life-threatening ventricular arrhythmias is higher than any other antiarrhythmic drug (7), and it has a lower risk of proarrhythmia than almost any of the other drugs (8). Its major disadvantage is the large number of side effects associated with its use. Pulmonary and hepatic toxicity, hypothyroidism, and hyperthyroidism are among the more serious problems; there are also neurologic, dermatologic, and ophthalmologic side effects. Careful monitoring of the patient, using serial blood tests, chest x-rays, and possibly pulmonary function tests, is necessary.

Implantable Cardioverter–Defibrillators

Implantable cardioverter–defibrillators (ICDs) for patients with life-threatening ventricular arrhythmias are highly effective in terminating ventricular tachycardia and fibrillation. The primary detection criterion for an ICD is rate; whenever the patient's heart rate exceeds the programmed value, a ventricular arrhythmia is presumed and therapy is delivered. There are additional detection features that may be added to the device program to discriminate between ventricular tachycardia and rapid atrial fibrillation or sinus tachycardia; but in general, ICDs function best with clear-cut differences between the patient's physiologic heart rates and the pathologic arrhythmia.

The majority of ICDs implanted today are third-generation devices, which not only deliver a shock to cardiovert or defibrillate but also provide antitachycardia pacing and backup bradycardia pacing (Fig. 8.4). The backup pacing available now is simple, fixed rate, ventricular pacing only. Antitachycardia pacing is useful for many patients with ventricular tachycardia, particularly those with more hemodynamically stable, slower forms of ventricular tachycardia. The majority of third-generation ICDs are implanted in the pectoral region, much like a permanent pacemaker.

An ICD can be excellent therapy in a patient who has survived a cardiac arrest or in any other patient who has infrequent episodes

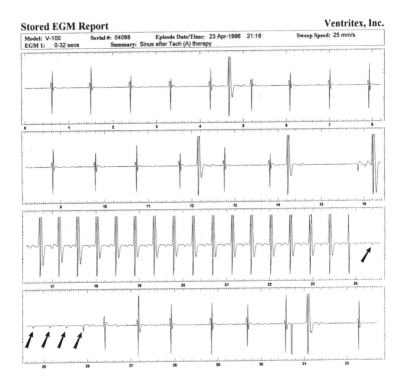

Figure 8.4: Intracardiac tracings retrieved from an ICD in a patient who had had therapy delivered for ventricular tachycardia. The **top two strips** show sinus rhythm with PVCs, the **third strip** shows sustained ventricular tachycardia, and the **bottom strip** shows the return to sinus rhythm. Ventricular tachycardia is terminated by antitachycardia pacing (*arrows*); signal is blanked out during pacing.

of hemodynamically compromising ventricular arrhythmia. If a patient has frequent episodes of well-tolerated ventricular tachycardia, a third-generation ICD is a good option as sole therapy only if the arrhythmia reliably terminates with pacing. Otherwise, patients typically require medical therapy with sotalol or amiodarone to reduce the frequency of shocks. Physicians must consider these issues when deciding on appropriate therapy for patients with ventricular tachycardia or fibrillation. Well-tolerated or minimally symptomatic arrhythmias may best be treated with antiarrhythmic drugs as the first line of therapy or even ignored. Furthermore, every effort must be made to optimize drug treatment of heart failure, including normalizing electrolyte abnormalities and correcting myocardial ischemia.

EVALUATION AND TREATMENT OF CARDIAC ARREST SURVIVORS

After a cardiac arrest, evaluation and treatment are essentially the same, regardless of the underlying cause of the heart disease (Fig. 8.5). After stabilization, the first issue is to determine whether there is a reversible cause for the arrest. Acute myocardial infarction, for example, is an obvious potential cause of cardiac arrest. Normally, cardiac arrest occurring within the first 48 h after myocardial infarction is ascribed to the infarction; and no further evaluation or treatment is necessary, unless there is a later recurrence. Circumstances become more confusing when a patient has a cardiac arrest requiring cardiopulmonary resuscitation, and a small creatine phosphokinase (CPK) rise occurs without ECG evidence of a transmural infarction. These cases should be treated as a primary arrhythmia. Electrolyte abnormalities such as hypokalemia or hypomagnesemia, hypoxia, severe heart failure, and the use of antiarrhythmic drugs may contrib-

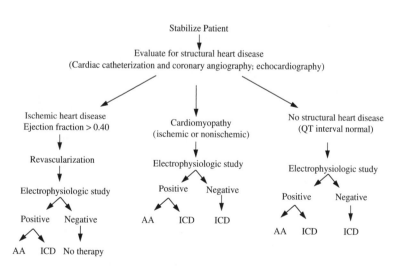

Figure 8.5:   Management of a patient after a cardiac arrest. *AA,* antiarrhythmic drugs.

ute to the pathogenesis of cardiac arrest, particularly in patients with poor ventricular function.

Many patients who have been resuscitated from cardiac arrest or who have hemodynamically compromising sustained ventricular tachycardia have no obvious identifiable cause for the arrhythmia aside from their clinically evident structural heart disease. If a patient has not undergone diagnostic cardiac catheterization previously, this will usually be done. It is critical to document CAD and determine the potential for mechanical revascularization. An alternative diagnostic approach may be an echocardiogram in conjunction with a noninvasive test for ischemia, such as an adenosine–thallium test.

With well-preserved ventricular function and high-grade coronary artery stenoses, treatment should be directed at relieving ischemia by angioplasty or bypass surgery (9). Specific treatment for arrhythmia may not be necessary. In such cases, clinicians often perform an electrophysiologic study after revascularization. Only if the patient has inducible ventricular arrhythmia after revascularization would most clinicians treat him or her with antiarrhythmic drugs or an ICD. On the other hand, patients with poor ventricular function typically remain at risk for life-threatening arrhythmia after revascularization and must be treated for their arrhythmia, regardless of other therapeutic procedures.

Most patients with documented ventricular tachycardia or fibrillation undergo electrophysiologic study (10). One exception may be patients whose cardiac arrest was documented to be the result of ventricular fibrillation. If an ICD is implanted, electrophysiologic testing can be accomplished through the device, making an antecedent study unnecessary.

If antiarrhythmic therapy is planned, then an electrophysiologic study should be done at baseline, unless therapy with amiodarone is planned and the patient is not a candidate for an ICD. If the presenting arrhythmia was a wide complex tachycardia, an electrophysiologic study at baseline can yield important information to help guide therapy. First, not all wide-complex tachycardias are ventricular tachycardias. If a patient actually has supraventricular tachycardia with aberration, the tachycardia may be curable with radiofrequency catheter ablation, and an ICD would clearly be inappropriate. Certain types of ventricular tachycardia are also curable with catheter ablation and may be identifiable only by electrophysiologic study. For example, right bundle branch re-entrant ventricular tachycardia, an unusual entity not well known except to electrophysiologists, has characteristic features that allow its identification at electrophysiologic study, is seen in patients with cardiomyopathies, and is curable by radiofrequency ablation of the right bundle branch (11).

Pacing techniques are used to provoke ventricular tachycardia in the laboratory, to confirm the diagnosis by intracardiac tracings, and to determine the hemodynamic stability of the arrhythmia. If a patient is conscious, it is usual to attempt to terminate the arrhythmia by overdrive pacing. Not only is this painless and effective in most cases but information can be obtained on the ease with which termination of the arrhythmia with antitachycardia pacing can be accomplished. Knowing that antitachycardia pacing is ineffective may sway a physician away from recommending a defibrillator for a relatively well-tolerated arrhythmia, if the only effective therapy that can be programmed is shock therapy.

After an initial electrophysiologic study, most patients require treatment with either antiarrhythmic drugs or an ICD. In the past, patients would often undergo serial trials with antiarrhythmic drugs, with repeat electrophysiologic testing after achieving steady-state drug levels. These long hospital stays are no longer feasible in today's medical climate. Just as important, however, is the fact that ICDs are much smaller and easier to implant now than in the past, when a thoracotomy was required, and ICD was a last resort. Today, ICDs are small enough to be implanted in the pectoral region, with a transvenous lead similar to a transvenous pacing electrode. With these changes, fewer antiarrhythmic drugs are tried, and relatively more ICDs are implanted.

Most clinicians often consider an initial trial of antiarrhythmic therapy in patients with ventricular tachycardia. If ventricular function is reasonably well preserved, clinicians generally use sotalol, with repeat electrophysiologic testing on a minimum dose of 160 mg twice a day (12). Repeat testing determines both efficacy and possible proarrhythmia. An optimal result is inability to provoke the arrhythmia on the antiarrhythmic drug; however, more difficult arrhythmia induction or slower and better-tolerated ventricular tachycardia may be acceptable. Proarrhythmia manifests as a faster, more unstable arrhythmia or one that is much easier to provoke (13). When proarrhythmia occurs, the arrhythmogenic drug should be discontinued and an alternative therapy chosen. For patients who have frequent ventricular arrhythmias on telemetry, suppression of the arrhythmia by antiarrhythmic drugs may give adequate evidence of a therapeutic effect (3). Most patients who have had life-threatening ventricular arrhythmias, however, do not have frequent enough arrhythmias on monitoring to guide therapy.

Most patients with serious ventricular dysfunction who require an antiarrhythmic drug receive amiodarone. It not only is probably the most effective agent available today but also has a low risk of proarrhythmia (8). It is usual to retest patients on amiodarone who could be candidates for an ICD, although this is controversial.

An important subset of patients have suffered a life-threatening ventricular arrhythmia but have no sustained ventricular arrhythmia on electrophysiologic testing. These patients may constitute 20 to 30% of those who have been resuscitated from a cardiac arrest. Since there is no way to assess efficacy of drug therapy in these patients, most receive ICDs.

PATIENTS WITH HIGH-GRADE VENTRICULAR ECTOPY WITHOUT SUSTAINED VENTRICULAR ARRHYTHMIAS

Ischemic Heart Disease

Patients with frequent ventricular arrhythmias after myocardial infarction have an increased risk of sudden death. The strong association has fostered a great deal of interest in finding ways to decrease this risk. The Cardiac Arrhythmia Suppression Trial (CAST), a well-known clinical trial, examined the role of the antiarrhythmic drugs flecainide, encainide, and moricizine in preventing sudden death in patients who had frequent ventricular ectopy after myocardial infarction (14). This prospective randomized study showed that treatment with antiarrhythmic drugs was associated with a threefold higher mortality than treatment with placebo. Since the drugs effectively reduced arrhythmia, it became clear that suppression of PVCs is not sufficient to lower the risk of sudden death in patients with ventricular arrhythmias after myocardial infarction.

An alternative approach to evaluation and treatment for these patients offers electrophysiologic study for risk stratification (Fig.

8.6). In the setting of chronic ischemic heart disease and an ejection fraction less than 0.40, a negative electrophysiologic study for ventricular tachycardia correlates well with absence of arrhythmic events in follow-up. In similar patients with inducible ventricular tachycardia, small nonrandomized studies have shown an apparent benefit from treatment with antiarrhythmic drugs that suppress the inducibility of the arrhythmia (15).

Two large-scale clinical trials have prospectively evaluated the value of treatment of such patients with antiarrhythmic drugs or ICDs. The Multicenter Unsustained Tachycardia Trial (MUSTT) is still in progress (16). This trial enrolls coronary disease patients with low ejection fraction and nonsustained ventricular tachycardia who have inducible sustained ventricular arrhythmias. Randomized treatment arms include antiarrhythmic drugs, ICDs, or no treatment; total mortality is the primary end point. The Multicenter Automatic Defibrillator Implantation Trial (MADIT) randomized patients with prior myocardial infarction, low ejection fraction, nonsustained ventricular tachycardia, and inducible ventricular tachycardia to treat-

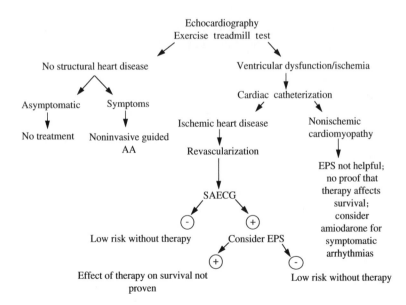

Figure 8.6: Management of a patient with nonsustained ventricular tachycardia. *AA,* antiarrhythmic drugs; *EPS,* electrophysiologic study; *SAECG,* signal-averaged ECG.

ment with antiarrhythmic drugs or an ICD. Preliminary results indicate a 54% reduction in total mortality in the patients with ICDs (17). These data were so compelling that the Food and Drug Administration recently gave approval for ICD implantation for this indication. Although the early MADIT results are certainly encouraging, we await the results of the MUSTT study for a definitive answer to this question.

Prophylactic use of amiodarone after myocardial infarction represents an alternative strategy. Two recent controlled trials—the Canadian Amiodarone Myocardial Infarction Arrhythmia Trial (CAMIAT) and the European Amiodarone Myocardial Infarction Trial (EMIAT)—suggested that amiodarone might decrease total mortality. Both trials were prospective, randomized, placebo-controlled trials of amiodarone therapy for survivors of acute myocardial infarction. CAMIAT enrolled patients 6 to 45 days after myocardial infarction who had more than 10 PVCs/h or any runs of ventricular tachycardia on a continuous electrocardiographic monitor. After a loading dose, patients received amiodarone at 200 to 400 mg/day or placebo. Amiodarone significantly reduced the incidence of arrhythmic death or resuscitation from ventricular fibrillation. Total mortality was slightly reduced with amiodarone, but the difference was not statistically significant. The results of the EMIAT study were similar.

Nonischemic

The appropriate treatment for patients with nonischemic cardiomyopathy and frequent PVCs or nonsustained ventricular tachycardia is even more uncertain than for coronary patients. In fact, no clear-cut correlation exists between the presence of ventricular arrhythmias in patients with nonischemic cardiomyopathies and risk for sudden death. Some studies have shown such a correlation, but others have shown that the presence of ventricular arrhythmias is associated with an increased risk for death from heart failure, not sudden death. Ventricular arrhythmias may provide a marker for severity of underlying heart disease, yet not for risk for arrhythmic death.

Electrophysiologic studies are notoriously unhelpful in patients with dilated nonischemic cardiomyopathy. Without a history of sustained ventricular arrhythmias, fewer than 10% of patients with nonischemic cardiomyopathy will have inducible sustained monomorphic ventricular tachycardia at electrophysiologic study (18). It is difficult to determine which patients are at risk for arrhythmic death and how therapy should be assessed.

Clinical studies of amiodarone therapy in patients with heart failure have yielded conflicting results. The Grupo de Estudio de la Sobrevida en la Insuficiencia Cardiaca en Argentina Trial (GESICA), found a 28% reduction in total mortality with amiodarone compared to placebo ($p = .024$) (19). Only 39% of the patients in this prospective, but nonblinded, study had CAD. In contrast, the Congestive Heart Failure Survival Trial Amiodarone CHF (CHF-Stat) (20) included patients with both ischemic and nonischemic cardiomyopathies, and all patients had frequent asymptomatic ventricular arrhythmias (at least 10 PVCs/h) but no history of sustained life-threatening arrhythmias. The dose of amiodarone was 400 mg/day the 1st year followed by 300 mg/day until the end of the study. After a median of 45 months, patients with nonischemic cardiomyopathies who were treated with amiodarone showed a trend toward improved survival, which did not reach statistical significance.

If a patient with dilated nonischemic cardiomyopathy and left ventricular dysfunction needs treatment for symptomatic ventricular arrhythmias, amiodarone should be the drug of choice. The risk of proarrhythmia from the other available antiarrhythmic drugs is increased in the setting of serious ventricular dysfunction.

AT RISK PATIENTS WITHOUT SYMPTOMS OR SERIOUS VENTRICULAR ECTOPY

Antiarrhythmic drug treatment has no role in the management of patients with serious ventricular dysfunction without apparent ventricular arrhythmias. However, since almost half of all patients with heart failure die suddenly, improving this statistic is an important goal. Survivors of a recent myocardial infarction should receive β-blockers if at all possible. Multiple clinical trials have shown improved survival with β-blockers (compared to treatment with placebo) after myocardial infarction (21). In patients with heart failure, β-blockers improve cardiac function and functional capacity and reduce the symptoms of heart failure. Carvedilol, which blocks both

α_1- and β_2-receptors, reduced mortality from both progressive heart failure as well as sudden death in patients with heart failure (22).

Treatment with angiotensin-converting enzyme (ACE) inhibitors improves survival in patients with congestive heart failure and in patients with reduced ventricular function after myocardial infarction (23). While total survival is improved, the effect of ACE-inhibiting vasodilators in preventing sudden death remains uncertain.

Other important factors may play a role in sudden death. Diuretics for heart failure may produce total body potassium depletion, despite potassium supplementation given to keep the serum potassium level normal. Digoxin doses should be adjusted and monitored appropriately, particularly with renal insufficiency. Optimal treatment for heart failure may minimize the chances that a serious arrhythmia will occur.

SUMMARY

Patients who have survived a serious ventricular arrhythmia with hemodynamic compromise must be evaluated for structural heart disease, and appropriate therapy must be instituted. Electrophysiologic studies are usually performed to evaluate the patient's arrhythmia substrate. Therapy can be either antiarrhythmic drugs, such as sotalol or amiodarone, or an ICD, depending on the arrhythmia and the clinical situation.

Patients who manifest nonsustained ventricular arrhythmias without sustained ventricular tachycardia or fibrillation are evaluated according to the underlying heart disease. In patients with ischemic heart disease, electrophysiologic study for risk stratification may have a role; this technique is under active clinical investigation. No conclusive evidence exists to support treatment with antiarrhythmic drugs or devices to enhance survival in patients with nonischemic cardiomyopathies.

Patients with heart failure who have ventricular arrhythmias should be treated optimally for their heart disease with the best current approaches to prolong survival.

REFERENCES
1. Nalos PC, Gang ES, Mandel WJ, et al. Utility of the signal-averaged electrocardiogram in patients presenting with sustained ventricular tachycardia or fibrillation while on an antiarrhythmic drug. Am Heart J 1988;115:108–114.

2. Gomes JA, Winters SL, Stewart D, et al. A new noninvasive index to predict sustained ventricular tachycardia and sudden death in the first year after myocardial infarction: based on signal averaged electrocardiogram, radionuclide ejection fraction and Holter monitoring. J Am Coll Cardiol 1987;10:349–357.

3. Mason JW. A comparison of electrophysiologic testing with Holter monitoring to predict antiarrhythmic drug efficacy for ventricular tachyarrhythmias. Electrophysiologic Study Versus Electrocardiographic Monitoring Investigators. N Engl J Med 1993;329:445–451.

4. Hohnloser SH, Woosley RL. Sotalol. N Engl J Med 1994;331:31–38.

5. Mason JW. A comparison of seven antiarrhythmic drugs in patients with ventricular tachyarrhythmias. Electrophysiologic Study Versus Electrocardiographic Monitoring Investigators. N Engl J Med 1993;329:452–458.

6. Kowey PR, Levine JH, Herre JM, et al. Randomized, double-blind comparison of intravenous amiodarone and bretylium in the treatment of patients with recurrent, hemodynamically destabilizing ventricular tachycardia or fibrillation. Intravenous Amiodarone Multicenter Investigators Group. Circulation 1995;92:3255–3263.

7. CASCADE Investigators. Randomized antiarrhythmic drug therapy in survivors of cardiac arrest (the CASCADE Study). Am J Cardiol 1993;72:280–287.

8. Gill J, Heel RC, Fitton A. Amiodarone: an overview of its pharmacological properties, and review of its therapeutic use in cardiac arrhythmias. Drugs 1992;43:69–110.

9. Kelly P, Ruskin JN, Vlahakes GJ, et al. Surgical coronary revascularization in survivors of prehospital cardiac arrest: its effect on inducible ventricular arrhythmias and long-term survival. J Am Coll Cardiol 1990;15:267–273.

10. Wilbur DJ, Garan H, Finkelstein D, et al. Out-of-hospital cardiac arrest: use of electrophysiologic testing in the prediction of long-term outcome. N Engl J Med 1988;318:19–24.

11. Caceres J, Jazayeri M, McKinnie J, et al. Sustained bundle branch reentry as a mechanism of clinical tachycardia. Circulation 1989;79:256–270.

12. Kehoe RF, Zheutlin TA, Dunnington CS, et al. Safety and efficacy of sotalol in patients with drug-refractory sustained ventricular tachyarrhythmias. Am J Cardiol 1990;65(Suppl):58A–64A.

13. Podrid PA. Aggravation of arrhythmia by antiarrhythmic drugs. In: Podrid PJ, Kowey PR, eds., Cardiac arrhythmia: mechanisms, diagnosis, and management. Baltimore, MD: Williams & Wilkins 1995:507–522.

14. Echt DS, Liebson PR, Mitchell LB, et al. Mortality and morbidity in patients receiving encainide, flecainide, or placebo: the Cardiac Arrhythmia Suppression Trial. N Engl J Med 1991;324:781–788.

15. Buxton AE, Marchlinski FE, Flores BT, et al. Nonsustained ventricular tachycardia in patients with coronary artery disease: role of electrophysiologic study. Circulation 1987;75:1178–1185.

16. Buxton AE, Fisher JD, Josephson ME, et al. Prevention of sudden death in patients with coronary artery disease: the Multicenter Unsustained Tachycardia Trial (MUSTT). Prog Cardiovasc Dis 1993;36:215–226.

17. Moss AJ, Hall WJ, Cannom DS, et al. Multicenter Automatic Defibrillator Implantation Trial (MADIT). Paper presented at the 17th Annual Scientific Sessions of the North American Society of Pacing and Electrophysiology, Seattle, May 1996.

18. Poll DS, Marchlinski FE, Buxton AE, Josephson ME. Usefulness of programmed stimulation in idiopathic dilated cardiomyopathy. Am J Cardiol 1986;58:992–997.

19. Doval HC, Nul DR, Grancelli HO, et al. Randomised trial of low-dose amiodarone in severe congestive heart failure. Grupo de Estudio de la Sobrevida en la Insuficiencia Cardiaca en Argentina (GESICA). Lancet 1994;344:493–498.

20. Singh SN, Fletcher RD, Fisher SG, et al. Amiodarone in patients with congestive heart failure and asymptomatic ventricular arrhythmia. Survival Trial of Antiarrhythmic Therapy in Congestive Heart Failure. N Engl J Med 1995;333:77–82.

21. Roberts R, Morris D, Pratt CM, Alexander RW. Pathophysiology, recognition, and treatment of acute myocardial infarction and its complications. In: Schlant RC, Alexander RW, eds., The heart, 8th ed., New York: McGraw-Hill, 1994:1162–1163.
22. Packer M, Bristow MR, Cohn JN, et al. The effect of carvedilol on morbidity and mortality in patients with chronic heart failure. U.S. Carvedilol Heart Failure Study Group. N Engl J Med 1996;334:1349–1355.
23. The SOLVD Investigators. Effect of enalapril on survival in patients with reduced left ventricular ejection fractions and congestive heart failure. N Engl J Med 1991;325:293–302.

SUGGESTED READING

Akhtar M. Clinical spectrum of ventricular tachycardia. Circulation 1990;82:1561–1573.

Brooks R, McGovern BA, Haran H, Ruskin JN. Current treatment of patients surviving out-of-hospital cardiac arrest. JAMA 1991;265:762–768.

Demirovic J, Myerburg RJ. Epidemiology of sudden coronary death: an overview. Prog Cardiovasc Dis 1994;37:39–48.

Gilman JK, Naccarelli GN. Sudden cardiac death. Curr Probl Cardiol 1992;17:693–778.

Stevenson WG, Stevenson LW, Middlekauff HR, Saxon LA. Sudden death prevention in patients with advanced ventricular dysfunction. Circulation 1993;88:2953–2961.

Chapter 9

Exercise Training

Randy W. Braith and Michael A. Welsch

Patients with chronic heart failure (CHF) uniformly complain of fatigue and activity intolerance. Tolerance for exercise, as assessed by peak oxygen consumption ($\dot{V}o_2$peak), is a powerful predictor of survival in these patients (Fig. 9.1). Before the 1980s, CHF patients were excluded from exercise rehabilitation programs because of concerns for safety. Previous treatment strategies maintained that rest was the first-line treatment for all stages and forms of CHF, and patients were advised to restrict physical activity to reduce circulatory demands. In acute or unstable CHF, rest can increase renal blood flow, enhance urine output, and augment pharmacologic diuresis. These changes improve hemodynamics and reduce ventricular volumes, both of which are beneficial in acute or unstable CHF. However, prolonged rest is neither necessary nor beneficial. In fact, similarity between the physiologic derangements of CHF and the changes seen with prolonged physical inactivity, or deconditioning, raises the possibility that deterioration of physical fitness may actually contribute to the secondary manifestations of CHF.

Over the past decade exercise rehabilitation has been used increasingly, with contemporary vasodilator drug therapy, to attain functional and symptomatic improvement in CHF. Aerobic exercise appears safe, once CHF patients have achieved clinical compensation. The risk of myocardial infarction or life-threatening arrhythmia in selected CHF patients is probably not significantly higher with exercise than with the background level of risk conferred by their heart failure.

This chapter reviews the factors contributing to exercise intolerance in patients with CHF and discusses the results of exercise rehabilitation studies in these patients. A summary of current recommendations and guidelines for exercise testing and exercise prescription is provided.

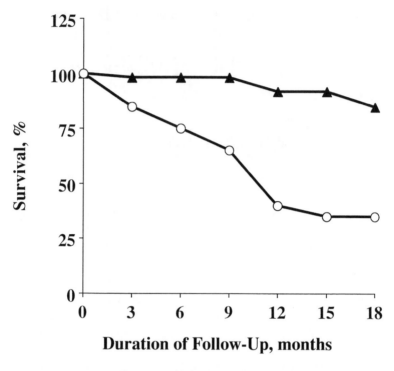

Figure 9.1:   Survival curves for heart failure patients with preserved exercise capacity (▲; group 1) and those with markedly impaired exercise capacity (O; group 2). Group 1: $n = 52$; age $= 47$ years; New York Heart Association (NYHA) class $= 3$; $\dot{V}O_2$peak $= 19.0$ mL/kg/min. Group 2: $n = 27$; age $= 53$ years; NYHA class $= 3$; $\dot{V}O_2$peak $= 10.5$ mL/kg/min. Modified from Mancini DM, Eisen H, Kussmaul W, et al. Value of peak exercise oxygen consumption for optimal timing of cardiac transplantation in ambulatory patients with heart failure. Circulation 1991;83:778–786.

FACTORS CONTRIBUTING TO EXERCISE INTOLERANCE IN CHF

CHF is a syndrome that encompasses abnormalities of both cardiac and noncardiac origin. Multiple peripheral compensatory adaptations, with short to long time constants, initially protect and assist the failing heart to maintain cardiac output and arterial pressure. These peripheral compensatory adaptations, including neuroendocrine, vascular, and skeletal muscle factors, may, however, ultimately contribute to marked exercise intolerance in CHF. Recent studies indicate that exercise training may reverse certain peripheral abnormalities present in CHF patients without significantly altering cardiac function. Thus exercise training may be an important, but underprescribed, adjunctive therapy in the treatment of CHF syndrome.

Impaired Left Ventricular Systolic Function

Central hemodynamic abnormalities are, by definition, the primary pathophysiologic features of CHF. Exercise tolerance, however, is not directly related to the degree of cardiac dysfunction. Left ventricular ejection fraction (LVEF) is important in assessing the extent of myocardial systolic dysfunction but is of little value in predicting an individual patient's ability to exercise. Similarly, LVEF during exercise is not a sensitive index for determining the beneficial effects of exercise rehabilitation in CHF. Both resting and exercise LVEF are essentially unchanged in CHF patients who successfully complete a program of endurance exercise training (1,2). Thus it is difficult to prove that the benefits of exercise rehabilitation programs for CHF patients can be attributed to improved myocardial function.

The weak relationship between LVEF and exercise tolerance in CHF has stimulated interest in peripheral mechanisms to explain exercise intolerance. The heart and the periphery, however, are closely coupled, both in healthy adults and in patients with CHF. A person's ability to use oxygen, measured as $\dot{V}o_2$peak, is closely related to maximal cardiac output; and cardiac output is related to exercise tolerance in patients with CHF (Fig. 9.2).

Impaired Left Ventricular Diastolic Function

CHF patients with preserved left ventricular (LV) systolic function also have significant exercise intolerance. In these patients, abnormalities in LV diastolic function prevent augmentation of stroke volume via the Frank–Starling mechanism; the result is severe exercise intolerance. One study reported that pulmonary capillary wedge pressures (PCWP) were markedly elevated at peak exercise in these patients compared with controls (26 versus 7 mm Hg) and $\dot{V}o_2$peak was reduced 48%, primarily owing to a 41% reduction in peak cardiac output (3). Increased LV filling pressure during exercise was not accompanied by increases in end-diastolic volume, indicating a restriction to LV filling. A recent study found significant improve-

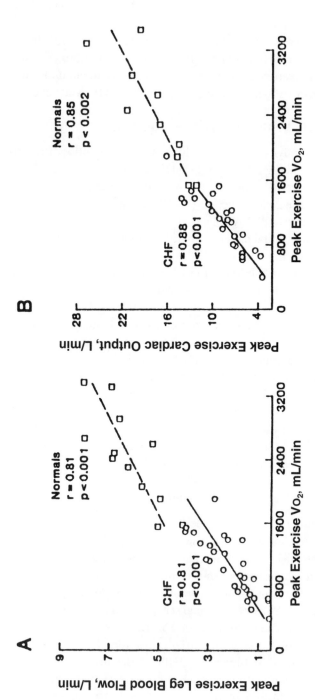

Figure 9.2: **A.** Relationship of Vo₂peak to cardiac output in 30 patients with CHF (O) caused by systolic ventricular dysfunction versus 12 controls (□). Modified from Sullivan MJ, Knight JD, Higginbotham MB, Cobb FR. **B.** Relation between central and peripheral hemodynamics during exercise in patients with chronic heart failure: muscle blood flow is reduced with maintenance of arterial perfusion pressure. Circulation 1989;80:769–781.

ment in $\dot{V}o_2$peak after exercise training in CHF patients with diastolic dysfunction caused by abnormal LV relaxation (4). However, patients with a restrictive pattern of diastolic dysfunction were unable to increase $\dot{V}o_2$peak.

Baroreflex Desensitization and Sympathetic Activation

In the acute phase of low-output CHF, arterial and cardiopulmonary baroreflexes are activated to help maintain systemic blood pressure. Sensitivity of both the arterial and the cardiopulmonary baroreceptors becomes diminished in CHF. The absence of baroreflex inhibitory input to medullary centers results in excessive sympathetic excitation. Plasma norepinephrine levels are twofold to threefold higher in CHF patients than in healthy controls (5), and direct microneurographic recordings also show dramatically increased levels of muscle sympathetic nerve activity (6). CHF patients become tachycardic with loss of heart rate variability, and peripheral vascular vasodilation is prevented by excessive sympathetic vasoconstrictor tone. The loss of baroreflex sensitivity and elevated levels of circulating norepinephrine are closely correlated with disease severity and overall survival (5,7).

Abnormal Stimulation of Neurohumoral Systems

The activation of neurohumoral fluid regulatory systems is the biochemical hallmark of CHF. Markedly elevated plasma renin activity, angiotensin II, aldosterone, arginine vasopressin, and atrial natriuretic peptide are associated with poor long-term prognosis in CHF (8). Activation of the renin–angiotensin–aldosterone axis has been attributed to low renal perfusion pressure, vasopressin is released as a result of combined stimuli from central osmoreceptors and peripheral baroreceptors, and atrial stretch is the most widely recognized stimulus for release of cardiac natriuretic peptides. These responses facilitate vasoconstriction and plasma volume expansion, which act to maintain forward cardiac output and systemic blood pressure. Sustained neurohumoral arousal, however, contributes to a further reduction in vasodilatory capacity.

Impaired Vasodilatory Capacity

Sympathetic stimulation and neurohumoral activation are potent sources of vasoconstriction in CHF. However, peripheral α-

adrenergic blockade (9) and angiotensin-converting enzyme (ACE) inhibitor therapy (10) do not immediately restore vasodilating capacity in CHF patients, indicating that intrinsic vascular abnormalities possibly contribute to impaired vasodilatory capacity. Currently, there are three mechanisms under investigation, all with long time constants, that help explain the vasodilatory impairment seen in CHF.

1. Vascular stiffness, caused by increased sodium and water content within vascular tissue, may be responsible for up to one-third of vasodilatory impairment in CHF (11). Acute diuretic therapy improves muscle blood flow but continued diuresis does not restore normal vasodilatory capacity, despite further reductions in fluid volume (11).
2. Chronic vascular deconditioning may also contribute to impaired vasodilatory capacity in CHF patients. Immobilization of the forearm is known to reduce vasodilatory capacity. Unilateral forearm exercise training, in contrast, was shown to significantly improve vasodilatory capacity, but only in the trained arm (12).
3. There is now compelling evidence of endothelial dysfunction in both peripheral and coronary vessels in patients with CHF (13,14). The consequence of endothelial dysfunction in CHF patients is increased endothelin 1, a powerful endothelium-derived vasoconstrictor, and reduced production of nitric oxide (NO), a potent endothelium-derived vasodilator. L-Arginine infusion (a precursor of NO) significantly improves vasodilation in CHF patients but not in controls, presumably by increasing NO synthesis (13). In contrast, nitroprusside infusion (NO donor directly to smooth muscle) elicits normal vasodilation in CHF patients, indicating that reduced vasodilatory capacity is owing to a defect in NO synthesis rather than a defect in vascular smooth muscle.

Skeletal Muscle Abnormalities

Exercise intolerance in CHF patients is often attributed to chronic underperfusion of exercising muscle. However, increasing blood supply to skeletal muscle does not result in an immediate improvement in $\dot{V}o_2$peak in these patients, indicating the presence of intrinsic abnormalities within the muscle that may be unrelated to blood flow. Skeletal muscle abnormalities include significant atrophy of oxidative type I muscle fibers, a marked decline in mitochondrial oxidative enzyme concentration and activity (succinate dehydrogenase, citrate synthase, cytochrome oxidase), and a reduction in mitochondrial volume and density (15).

The cross-sectional area of the thigh, as measured by MRI, is reduced by 13 to 15% in CHF patients. The mechanism for muscle atrophy in CHF patients is unclear but has been linked to malnutrition, deconditioning, increased catabolism owing to sympathetic hyperactivity, increased serum cortisol, and tumor necrosis factor. It should be noted, however, that muscle mass is weakly correlated with $\dot{V}o_2$peak in CHF patients, suggesting that muscle size contributes only modestly to exercise intolerance (16).

Muscle biopsies obtained from CHF patients show that atrophy is more pronounced in highly oxidative, fatigue resistant, type I muscle fibers (15). Selective atrophy of type I fibers results in a shift in fiber type distribution toward the glycolytic, less fatigue resistant, type II muscle fibers. These morphologic changes are thought to contribute to diminished exercise tolerance and decreased $\dot{V}o_2$peak.

Pulmonary Abnormalities

Exertional dyspnea is a prominent symptom in CHF and a variety of abnormalities in pulmonary function are believed to be exacerbated by CHF. Traditionally, exertional dyspnea was attributed to exaggerated increases in left ventricular filling pressure and corresponding PCWP; however, recent hemodynamic studies have failed to correlate dyspnea symptoms with measurements of PCWP (17). Dyspnea in nonedematous CHF patients may be as much or more related to deconditioning and abnormalities in the metabolism of exercising skeletal muscle than to pulmonary congestion. In a group of CHF patients studied before and after exercise training, PCWP was unchanged by training, despite a 23% increase in exercise capacity and a reduction in dyspnea symptoms (17).

A recent study performed spirometry and measured pulmonary diffusion capacity in patients immediately before and after cardiac transplantation to determine the impact of CHF on pulmonary function (18). Abnormalities on spirometry were completely reversible with normalization of cardiovascular physiologic processes after transplantation. The restrictive pulmonary defects were attributed to encroachment by the enlarged heart. However, abnormal pulmonary diffusing capacity observed in CHF patients before transplantation was not resolved and persisted following transplantation, with or without restrictive or obstructive pulmonary defects (Fig. 9.3).

Respiratory muscle fatigue also contributes to dyspnea in CHF patients. A study using near-infrared spectroscopy to monitor accessory respiratory muscle perfusion found exercise-induced deoxygen-

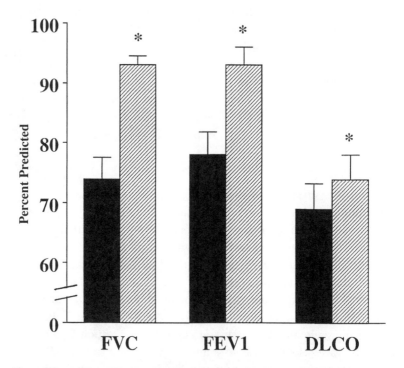

Figure 9.3:   Forced vital capacity (*FVC*), forced expired volume in 1 s (*FEV₁*), and pulmonary diffusing capacity (*DLCO*) in 11 patients before (*solid bars*) and after (*hatched bars*) cardiac transplantation. Values represent the mean plus or minus SEM. Significance: * $p \leq .05$. Modified from Braith RW, Limacher MC, Leggett SH, et al. Exercise-induced hypoxemia in heart transplant recipients. J Am Coll Cardiol 1993;22:768–776.

ation of accessory respiratory muscles in patients with CHF, implying that decreased cardiac output during exercise results in deoxygenation of accessory respiratory muscles (19).

RESPONSES TO EXERCISE TRAINING

The few training studies in patients with CHF and mild to moderate LV dysfunction are limited by small samples and young populations that consist predominantly of men with coronary disease. To date, all published exercise training studies in CHF patients have been performed with medically stable patients—New York Heart Association (NYHA) classes I to III—with a functional capacity greater than 14 mL/kg/min or 4 METS. Despite these limitations, early observational studies that lead to the concerns regarding the dangers of exercise training for all CHF patients are being superseded by randomized controlled trials using the latest methods of documentation.

The first report indicating that CHF patients could safely participate in and benefit from an exercise rehabilitation program did not appear until 1979 (20). A total of 18 post–myocardial infarction patients with an average LVEF of 18% trained at 70 to 85% of maximal heart rate for 20 to 45 min, 4 days/week. The beneficial effect of exercise training was improved time to exhaustion on the treadmill, without any untoward cardiac events. Since that early study, six randomized controlled trials (21–26), four nonrandomized controlled studies (27–30), and three observational studies (1,31,32) have been reported. The studies vary considerably in the duration, intensity, and length of exercise training; but a consistent finding is that CHF patients can improve functional capacity through exercise training, without increasing the risk for cardiovascular complications.

Despite the consistent results from training studies, the mechanism(s) underlying the beneficial effects of exercise training in CHF patients remain unclear. It has been clearly demonstrated, however, that the increases in exercise capacity are related to reversing the peripheral abnormalities rather than improving cardiac function.

Peak Oxygen Consumption

Training-induced improvements in $\dot{V}o_2peak$ are a consistent finding in CHF patients and range from 1.4 to 7 mL/kg/min (1,31,33).

One study reported a 23% increase in $\dot{V}o_2$peak (from 16.8 to 20.6 mL/kg/min) in CHF patients (LVEF 24 ± 10%) after 4 months of exercise training consisting of 4 h of monitored exercise per week (1). There were no changes in rest or exercise PCWP, stroke volume, or LVEF. Researchers at the University of Florida found a 26% increase in $\dot{V}o_2$peak in CHF patients (ischemic disease, NYHA class II or III, LVEF 30%, age 54 to 68 years) who participated in a program of supervised treadmill walking 3 days/week for 16 weeks at 40 to 70% of $\dot{V}o_2$peak (33) (Fig. 9.4). Walking time to exhaustion during a modified Naughton treadmill protocol was also significantly increased by 30% in the training group.

CHF patients with less than 40% LVEF and anginal symptoms on a treadmill test may not achieve exercise training–induced improvements in $\dot{V}o_2$peak, because the low anginal threshold could limit the exercise training intensity (31). However, patients whose LVEF is less than 40% after a recent large myocardial anterior myocardial infarction can safely engage in an exercise program and increase their $\dot{V}o_2$peak if they remain free of ischemia (31).

Cardiac Function

Despite consistent findings of improved $\dot{V}o_2$peak, cardiac output shows either no change (1) or a very small increase (2) after a program of exercise training in CHF patients. One study asked CHF patients to exercise for 60 min, 3 to 5 days/week at 75% of peak heart rate (HR) (1). Cardiac output (and LVEF) was not changed by 16 to 24 weeks of training. In contrast, a randomized 8-week crossover study comparing exercise training and restriction of training in 11 CHF patients reported an increase in both submaximal and maximal cardiac output during supine bicycle exercise (2). Increased submaximal cardiac output (25 W) was attributed to changes in stroke volume with no change in heart rate. The increase in cardiac output at peak exercise intensity was the result of increased peak heart rate and the ability of CHF patients to exercise at a greater absolute work load.

There is no evidence that exercise training in CHF patients improves left ventricular function, as defined by LVEF. One nonrandomized controlled study reported a significant post-training deterioration in LVEF and increase in LV asynergy in CHF patients with

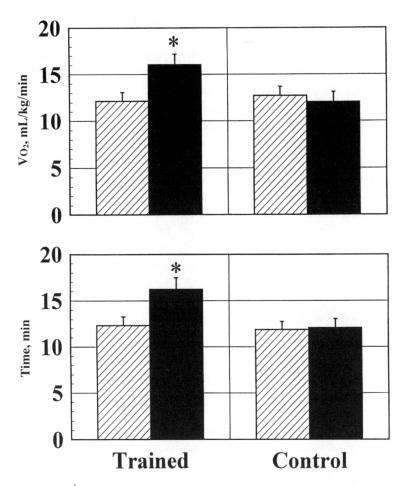

Figure 9.4: $\dot{V}_{O_2}$peak and treadmill time to exhaustion in heart failure patients before (*hatched bars*) and after (*solid bars*) 16 weeks of exercise training (*trained; n* = 14) or a control period (*control; n* = 14). Values represent the mean plus or minus the SEM. Significance: * $p \leq$ .05. Modified from Kluess HA, Welsch MA, Properzio AM, et al. Accelerated skeletal muscle recovery following exercise training in heart failure. Circulation 1996;94(Suppl):I192.

anterior myocardial infarction (28). Subsequent studies, however, have not confirmed those findings (24–26,29,30). A recent multicenter randomized trial was designed to determine the effects of exercise on LV remodeling in patients recovering from anterior myocardial infarction (26). The 6-month training program consisted of aggressive stationary cycling and walking. Although patients with an LVEF of less than 40% had greater ventricular enlargement before training, they did not have further enlargement or deterioration after training.

Another recent exercise training study used restriction (to anterior myocardial infarctions), stratification (by LVEF ≤ 30% and >30%), and a controlled randomized design to overcome biases that have plagued most earlier exercise studies (24). Reliable and validated radionuclide ventriculography and echocardiography were used to assess LV function before and after training. The results substantiate the conclusion that exercise is safe for patients with LV dysfunction after myocardial infarction. In aggregate, the experience to date indicates that selected CHF patients without clinical complications can benefit from exercise training without negative effects on ventricular size and topography.

Baroreflex and Sympathetic Activation

Markers of autonomic nervous system function in CHF patients, including, resting heart rate, RR variability, and whole-body radiolabeled norepinephrine spillover, show a significant shift away from sympathetic activity to greater dominance of vagal parasympathetic tone after a program of exercise training (1,2). A consistent response to exercise training in CHF patients is a reduction in resting heart rate, reflecting the shift in autonomic nervous system balance away from sympathetic influence. These findings are particularly intriguing since sympathetic hyperactivity, elevated resting heart rate, and chronotropic incompetence are factors that affect survival in CHF patients.

One study found a 30% improvement in baroreflex sensitivity in 70 CHF patients following a program of exercise training (7). Improved baroreceptor sensitivity was correlated with decreased sympathetic and neurohumoral activation and an increase in parasympathetic activity and heart rate variability. The clinical implication is that improved baroreflex function and vagal tone could diminish susceptibility to life-threatening arrhythmias in CHF patients.

Neurohumoral Systems

A recent study at the University of Florida was the first to measure fluid regulatory hormone levels in CHF patients immediately before and after 4 months of exercise training to determine the effect of exercise rehabilitation on neurohumoral hyperactivity (34). A total of 19 CHF patients (ischemic disease; NYHA class II or III) were randomly assigned to a training group ($n = 10$; age 55 to 67 years; EF $= 30 \pm 6\%$) or to a control group that did not train ($n = 9$; age = 55 to 69 years; EF $= 29 \pm 7\%$). Exercise consisted of supervised walking three times per week for 16 weeks at 40 to 70% of peak oxygen uptake. Before training, values for angiotensin II, aldosterone, vasopressin, and atrial natriuretic peptide did not differ between the groups (Fig. 9.5). After training, all rest neurohormone

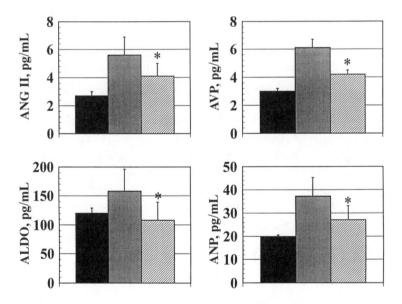

Figure 9.5: Rest plasma levels of angiotensin II (*ANG II*), aldosterone (*ALDO*), arginine vasopressin (*AVP*), and atrial natriuretic peptide (*ANP*) in age-matched untrained healthy controls (*solid bars; n* = 11) and heart failure patients (*n* = 10) before (*shaded bars*) and after (*hatched bars*) 16 weeks of exercise training. Values represent the mean plus or minus the SEM. Significance: * $p \le .05$ versus pretraining. Modified from Braith RW, Feigenbaum MS, Welsch MA, et al. Neuroendocrine hyperactivity in heart failure is buffered by endurance exercise. Circulation 1996; 94(Suppl):I192.

levels were significantly reduced by approximately 30% in the exercise group but unchanged in the control group. This training adaptation likely reflects increased baroreflex sensitivity and could contribute to the reduction in clinically significant cardiac events in CHF patients.

Vasodilatory Capacity

Hornig et al. (13) were the first to suggest that an exercise program can enhance vasodilatory capacity in patients with CHF. In their crossover trial, patients participated in 4 weeks of daily handgrip exercise at 70% of maximal voluntary contraction. High-resolution ultrasound was used to measure radial artery diameter during reactive hyperemia (endothelium-dependent dilation) and during sodium nitroprusside infusion (endothelium-independent dilation). Exercise training restored flow-dependent vasodilatory capacity in CHF patients, suggesting training-induced stimulation of endothelial NO synthesis. It should be noted that enhanced vasodilation was specific to the region trained and was lost after 6 weeks of cessation of training.

Short-term vasodilator therapy does not have an immediately favorable effect on $\dot{V}o_2peak$, despite effective pharmacologic blockade of the vasoconstrictor systems and acute hemodynamic benefits (10). Instead, benefits accrue slowly during the 2 to 12 weeks following therapy. A study comparing placebo with ACE inhibitor treatment—with and without exercise training—showed the greatest improvement in symptomatic status and lowest rate to pressure product in CHF patients with a combination of ACE inhibitor treatment and exercise training, suggesting a role for chronic peripheral adaptations in this response (23).

Skeletal Muscle Metabolism

Three studies in CHF patients have reported significant improvement in metabolic capacity following short-term exercise training programs (35–37). The studies all used ^{31}P-NMR spectroscopy and in-magnet exercise protocols to assess the effects of training on muscle bioenergetics. Muscle endurance was increased up to 260% without any change in muscle mass, limb blood flow, and cardiac output (35). Instead, improved exercise tolerance was attributed to reduced depletion of phosphocreatine (PCr), higher muscle pH at submaximal work loads, and more rapid resynthesis of PCr, which is an indicator of mitochondrial oxidative phosphorylation (36,37).

Researchers at the University of Florida recently completed the longest randomized controlled exercise trial in CHF patients to determine if a training program would provide an adequate stimulus to reverse the skeletal muscle abnormalities present in many patients with CHF (33). Muscle metabolism was assessed by ^{31}P-NMR spectroscopy in the medial head of the gastrocnemius before and after a 4-month walking program. The in-magnet exercise protocol consisted of repetitive plantar flexion at a low-intensity (25% of maximal voluntary contraction) and high-intensity (85%) work load. The results from this study show a marked reduction (19%) in the inorganic phosphate (P_i) to phosphocreatine ratio (P_i:PCr) during the low-intensity exercise and a significant decrease (30%) in intramuscular deproteinated inorganic phosphate (H_2PO_4) during the high-intensity exercise (Fig. 9.6).

The 19% reduction in P_i:PCr during the low-intensity exercise protocol is thought to reflect an improved capacity of exercising muscle to produce ATP from oxidative metabolic pathways. The 30% reduction in H_2PO_4 may have contributed to the significant improvement in exercise time to exhaustion, because H_2PO_4 accumulation interferes with the contractile apparatus (Fig. 9.6). In addition, exercise training resulted in a significant improvement (28%) in PCr resynthesis following both the low- and high-intensity protocols, indicating improved recovery kinetics. In contrast, the skeletal muscle metabolic profile remained unchanged in the control group.

Although the precise mechanism for improved muscle energetics, as determined by ^{31}P-NMR spectroscopy, are not fully understood, the reduced P_i:PCr and increased PCr resynthesis likely reflects either an increase in the number of mitochondria, an increase in enzyme activity, or an improved ability to shuttle hydrolysis products across the mitochondrial membranes. The clinical implications from recent ^{31}P-NMR spectroscopy studies is that exercise training may serve as a significant stimulus to reverse certain skeletal muscle metabolic abnormalities in patients with CHF.

Summary of Responses to Exercise Training

Exercise training increases functional capacity and improves symptoms in selected patients with compensated stable CHF and

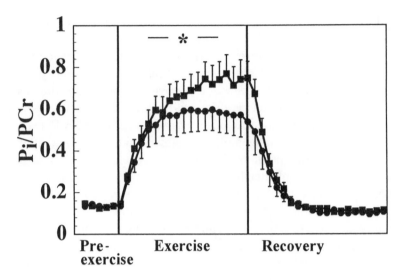

Figure 9.6: The P_i:PCr before, during, and immediately following low-intensity plantar flexion (25% maximal voluntary contraction) in heart failure patients ($n = 14$) before (■) and after (●) 16 weeks of exercise training. The P_i:PCr ratio, as determined by ^{31}P-NMR spectroscopy, is an index of skeletal muscle oxidative capacity. Values represent the mean plus or minus the SEM. Significance: * $p \leq .05$. Modified from Kluess HA, Welsch MA, Properzio AM, et al. Accelerated skeletal muscle recovery following exercise training in heart failure. Circulation 1996;94(Suppl):I192.

moderate to severe LV systolic dysfunction. These favorable outcomes usually occur without deterioration in LV function. Peripheral adaptations, particularly in skeletal muscle and peripheral circulation, appear to mediate the improvement in exercise tolerance rather than adaptations in the cardiac musculature. Patients who have a combination of LV dysfunction and residual myocardial ischemia, however, may not benefit from exercise training. Exercise training appears to optimize the symptomatic and functional benefits of ACE inhibitor therapy. The most consistent benefits occur with exercise training at least three times per week for 12 or more weeks. The duration of aerobic exercise training sessions can vary from 20 to 40 min, at an intensity of 70 to 85% of peak HR on the graded exercise test or 40 to 60% of $\dot{V}o_2$peak.

DESIGNING AN EXERCISE PROGRAM

Risk Stratification and Patient Screening

Recently, the American Heart Association (AHA), the American College of Sports Medicine, the American Association for Cardiovascular and Pulmonary Rehabilitation, and the Centers for Disease Control and Prevention have published updated guidelines, standards, and position statements on exercise in clinical populations (38). These organizations uniformly encourage stratification of individuals into risk categories before encouraging them to engage in an exercise program. Using these risk strata, the AHA recommends that medically stable CHF patients may participate in exercise training programs. The majority of stable CHF patients will be class C patients; but a significant number of patients with mild heart failure may be considered class B (i.e., an exercise capacity of 6 METS and an LVEF of 40 to 60%) and be qualified to participate in comprehensive rehabilitation programs, including light to moderate resistance training. Regardless of the classification, the exercise program should be individualized and medical supervision provided until safety is established.

Before starting an exercise program, CHF patients must be in stable condition and fluid volume status should be controlled. CHF patients with an LVEF of less than 30% should be carefully screened for ischemia. Pretraining evaluation with a symptom-limited bicycle or treadmill graded exercise test is essential. Only patients free of unstable or exercise-induced ventricular arrhythmias should be considered for exercise training. In addition, echocardiographic assessment of ventricular function and expired gas analysis for assessment of $\dot{V}o_2peak$ are helpful in preparing specific exercise prescription guidelines concerning the frequency, intensity, duration, mode, and progression of the exercise program. The selection process is summarized in Figure 9.7.

Initial Exercise Intensity

The initial exercise intensity should be customized for each patient. Because many CHF patients have marked exercise intolerance, it may be necessary to use an interval training approach, with 2 to

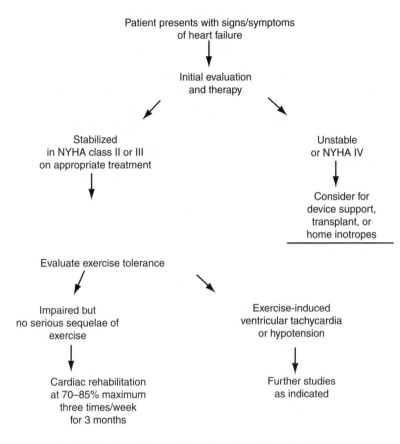

Figure 9.7: Selection of CHF patients for cardiac rehabilitation.

6 min of low-level activities alternated with 1- to 2-min rest periods. The frequency of training may be as much as two to three times/ day during the early stages of the program, with symptoms and general fatigue serving as guidelines to determine frequency. Warmup and cooldown periods should be longer than normal. Determination of appropriate exercise intensity for CHF patients should be based on $\dot{V}o_2$peak rather than HR peak because the chronotropic response to exercise is frequently abnormal in CHF patients.

A starting exercise intensity of 40 to 60% of $\dot{V}o_2$peak is recommended. Alternatively, the initial exercise intensity should be 10 beats below any significant symptoms, including, angina, exertional hypotension, dysrhythmias, and dyspnea. Continuous supervision may be necessary during the early stages of the exercise program for all CHF patients, and frequent monitoring of blood pressure and echocardiographic responses should be used in CHF patients at higher risk (AHA class C). Rating of perceived exertion should range from 11 to 14 (light to somewhat hard) on the 6 to 20 category Borg perceived exertion scale. Anginal symptoms should not exceed 2+ on the 0 to 4 angina scale (moderate to bothersome), and exertional dyspnea should not exceed 2+ on the dyspnea scale (mild, some difficulty) (38). Initially, full resuscitation equipment should be available.

Exercise Program Progression

The duration of exercise should be gradually increased to 30 min as tolerated by the patient. In selected patients, after a prolonged period (6 to 12 weeks) of supervised exercise sessions without evidence of adverse events or arrhythmia, submaximal exercise may continue away from the supervised environment (e.g., a home program). The choice of exercise should be predominantly cardiovascular in nature, such as walking and cycling. Current guidelines by the AHA and other exercise science organizations do not include recommendations for a resistance training component for CHF patients. However, light to moderate resistance training could be integrated as part of a comprehensive rehabilitation program for low-risk (AHA class B) CHF patients who have successfully completed 6 to 12 weeks of cardiovascular exercise training without adverse events.

SUMMARY

New standards and guidelines have been directed toward physicians and other health professionals who are involved in regular exercise testing and exercise training (39). For primary care physicians, who are increasingly using exercise testing, clinical competency requirements are available (39).

Rehabilitation personnel must watch for symptoms of cardiac decompensation during exercise, including cough or dyspnea, hypotension, lightheadedness, cyanosis, angina, and arrhythmias. Patients' body weight should be recorded before exercise, and daily pulmonary auscultation for rales and shortness of breath is recommended. Patients should avoid exercise immediately after eating or taking a vasodilator. Fluid and electrolyte balance is vital. Patients who have potassium or magnesium deficiency should take supplements to replenish electrolytes before embarking on an exercise program.

REFERENCES

1. Sullivan MJ, Higginbotham MB, Cobb FR. Exercise training in patients with severe left ventricular dysfunction: hemodynamic and metabolic effects. Circulation 1988;78:506–515.
2. Coats AJ, Adamopoulos S, Radaelli A, et al. Controlled trial of physical training in chronic heart failure: exercise performance, hemodynamics, ventilation, and autonomic function. Circulation 1992;85:2119–2131.
3. Kitzman DW, Higginbotham MB, Cobb FR, et al. Exercise intolerance in patients with heart failure and preserved left ventricular systolic function: failure of the Frank-Starling mechanism. J Am Coll Cardiol 1991;17:1065–1072.
4. Belardinelli R, Georgiou D, Cianci G, et al. Exercise training improves left ventricular diastolic filling in patients with dilated cardiomyopathy: clinical and prognostic implications. Circulation 1995;91:2775–2784.
5. Cohn JN, Levine TB, Olivari MT, et al. Plasma norepinephrine as a guide to prognosis in patients with chronic congestive heart failure. N Engl J Med 1984;311:819–823.
6. Leimbach WN, Wallin G, Victor RG, et al. Direct evidence from intraneuronal recordings for increased central sympathetic outflow in patients with heart failure. Circulation 1986;73:913–919.
7. La Rovere MT, Mortara A, Specchia G, Schwartz PJ. Myocardial infarction and baroreflex sensitivity: clinical studies. J Ital Cardiol 1992;22:639–645.
8. Levine TB, Francis GS, Goldsmith SR, et al. Activity of the sympathetic nervous system and renin–angiotensin system assessed by plasma hormone levels and their relationship to hemodynamic abnormalities in heart failure. Am J Cardiol 1982;49:1659–1666.
9. LeJemtel T, Maskin C, Lucido D, Chadwick B. Failure to augment maximal limb blood flow in response to one-leg versus two-leg exercise in patients with severe heart failure. Circulation 1986;74:245–251.
10. Drexler H, Banhardt U, Meinertz T, et al. Contrasting peripheral short-term and long-term effects of converting enzyme inhibition in patients with congestive heart failure. Circulation 1989;79:491–502.
11. Sinoway LI, Minotti J, Musch T, et al. Enhanced metabolic vasodilation secondary to diuretic therapy in decompensated congestive heart failure secondary to coronary artery disease. Am J Cardiol 1987;60:107–111.
12. Sinoway L, Shenberger J, Wilson J, et al. A 30-day forearm work protocol increases maximal forearm blood flow. J Appl Physiol 1987;62:1063–1067.
13. Hirooka Y, Imaizumi T, Harada S, et al. Endothelium-dependent forearm vasodilation with acetylcholine but not that with substance P is impaired in patients with heart failure. J Cardiovasc Pharmacol 1992;20:S221–S225.
14. Hornig B, Maier V, Drexler H. Physical training improves endothelial function in patients with chronic heart failure. Circulation 1996;93:210–214.
15. Drexler H, Reide U, Munzel T, et al. Alterations of skeletal muscle in chronic heart failure. Circulation 1992;85:1751–1759.
16. Mancini DM, Walter G, Reichek N, et al. Contribution of skeletal muscle atrophy to exercise intolerance and altered muscle metabolism in heart failure. Circulation 1992;85:1364–1373.

17. Sullivan MJ, Higginbotham MB, Cobb FR. Exercise training in patients with chronic heart failure delays ventilatory anaerobic threshold and improves submaximal exercise performance. Circulation 1989;79:324–329.
18. Braith RW, Limacher MC, Leggett SH, et al. Exercise-induced hypoxemia in heart transplant recipients. J Am Coll Cardiol 1993;22:768–776.
19. Mancini DM, Henson D, LaManca J, Levine S. Respiratory muscle function and dyspnea in patients with chronic congestive heart failure. Circulation 1992;86: 909–918.
20. Lee AP, Ice R, Blessey R, Sanmarco ME. Long-term effects of physical training on coronary patients with impaired LV function. Circulation 1979;60:1519–1526.
21. Sullivan MJ, Knight JD, Higginbotham MB, Cobb FR. Relation between central and peripheral hemodynamics during exercise in patients with chronic heart failure: muscle blood flow is reduced with maintenance of arterial perfusion pressure. Circulation 1989;80:769–781.
22. Grodzinski E, Jette M, Blumchen G, Borer JS. Effects of a four-week training program on left ventricular function as assessed by radionuclide ventriculography. J Cardiopulm Rehab 1987;7:518–524.
23. Meyer TR, Casadei B, Coats AJ, et al. Angiotensin-converting enzyme inhibition and physical training in heart failure. J Intern Med 1991;230:407–413.
24. Jette M, Heller R, Landry F, Blumchen G. Randomized 4-week program in patients with impaired left ventricular function. Circulation 1991;84:1561–1567.
25. Giannuzzi P, Temporelli PL, Tavazzi L, et al. EAMI-exercise training in anterior myocardial infarction: an ongoing multicenter randomized study: preliminary results on left ventricular function and remodeling. Chest 1992;101(Suppl 5):315S–321S.
26. Giannuzzi P, Tavazzi L, Temporelli PL, et al. Long-term physical training and left ventricular remodeling after anterior myocardial infarction: results of the Exercise in Anterior Myocardial Infarction (EAMI) Trial. J Am Coll Cardiol 1993;22:1821–1829.
27. Conn EH, Willeams RS, Wallace AG. Exercise responses before and after physical conditioning in patients with severely depressed LV function. Am J Cardiol 1982;49:296–300.
28. Jugdutt BI, Michorowski BL, Kappagoda CT. Exercise training after anterior Q wave myocardial infarction: importance of regional left ventricular function and topography. J Am Coll Cardiol 1988;12:362–372.
29. Hedback B, Perk J. Can high-risk patients after myocardial infarction participate in comprehensive cardiac rehabilitation? Scand J Rehab Med 1990;22:15–20.
30. Hertzeanu HL, Shemesh J, Aron LA, et al. Ventricular arrhythmias in rehabilitated and nonrehabilitated post-myocardial patients with left ventricular dysfunction. Am J Cardiol 1993;71:24–27.
31. Arvan S. Exercise performance of the high risk acute myocardial infarction patient after cardiac rehabilitation. Am J Cardiol 1988;62:197–201.
32. Kellerman JJ, Shemesh J, Fisman EZ, et al. Arm exercise training in the rehabilitation of patients with impaired ventricular function and heart failure. Cardiology 1990;77:130–138.
33. Kluess HA, Welsch, MA, Properzio AM, et al. Accelerated skeletal muscle recovery following exercise training in heart failure. Circulation 1996;94(Suppl): I192.
34. Braith RW, Feigenbaum MS, Welsch MA, et al. Neuroendocrine hyperactivity in heart failure is buffered by endurance exercise. Circulation 1996;94(Suppl):I192.
35. Minotti J, Johnson E, Hudson et al. Training-induced skeletal muscle adaptations are independent of systemic adaptations. J Appl Physiol 1990;68:289–294.
36. Adamopoulos S, Coats A, Brunothe F. Physical training improves skeletal muscle metabolism in patients in chronic heart failure. J Am Coll Cardiol 1992;21:1101–1106.

37. Stratton J, Dunn J, Adamopoulos S, et al. Training partially reverses skeletal muscle metabolic abnormalities during exercise in heart failure. J Appl Physiol 1994;76:1575–1582.
38. American College of Sports Medicine. Guidelines for exercise testing and prescription, 5th ed., Baltimore, MD: Williams & Wilkins, 1995.
39. Braith RW, Mills RM. Exercise training in patients with congestive heart failure: how to achieve benefits safely. Postgrad Med 1994;96:119–130.

Section 2

Providers and Their Roles in Patient Care

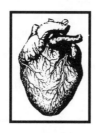

Chapter 10

Continuing Care of the Heart Failure Patient

Roger M. Mills Jr.

Throughout this book, the authors have emphasized a team approach to caring for the patient with heart failure. In today's health care environment, two or more physicians may be involved in leadership. This chapter addresses some of the issues involved when both a primary care physician and a specialist in cardiology share in the care of a single patient. Like many other difficult situations, the sharing of responsibility requires communication. Both physicians must share information and agree on who will do what. The suggestions offered in this chapter have worked in large referral practices in the U.S. South and the Midwest; but they are given as only guidelines to highlight issues, not as iron-clad rules.

What works for two physicians may vary with locale, with the nature of their practices, and with the reimbursement system in which they operate. Table 10.1 outlines the division of effort that my group has empirically developed.

SPECIALTY CARE ISSUES IN HEART FAILURE

The cardiologists who manage heart failure patients may provide a variety of services to different patients, from essentially primary care to purely consultation. Nonetheless, the cardiologist has some responsibilities that are unique and clearly different from those of the primary physician, including the following.

1. *Make a complete and accurate diagnosis.* The cardiologist should employ appropriate diagnostic technology to define the etiologic, anatomic, and physiologic aspects of the

Table 10.1.   Division of Responsibilities between Primary and Specialty Care Physicians

Primary Care	Specialist
• Assess disability	• Ensure complete diagnostic evaluation
• Evaluate social support systems	• Consider surgical management
• Educate other caregivers	• Pursue electrophysiologic evaluations
• Foster rehabilitation	• Maximize medical therapy
• Manage emotional consequences of heart disease	• Consider transplantation

patient's cardiovascular disease and to assess functional capacity.

2. *Actively consider the role of surgical intervention for each patient.* As clinical data confirming the benefits of revascularization for patients with impaired ventricular function or advanced valvular disease continue to accumulate, the consulting cardiologist should consider surgical intervention and document the discussion of the risks and benefits of surgery for most patients.

3. *Aggressively pursue electrophysiologic stability.* In heart failure, almost half of all deaths are sudden, and rhythm disturbances are part and parcel of the clinical syndrome. Recent data indicate significantly better survival in patients with symptomatic ventricular arrhythmia managed with implantable cardioverter–defibrillator devices and marked symptomatic improvement in patients with chronic atrial fibrillation who undergo AV nodal ablation and implantation of a permanent (VVI-R) pacemaker. These observations mandate screening almost all heart failure patients for electrophysiologic stability and aggressively managing those who have significant arrhythmia.

4. *Document functional status and consider transplantation.* Given the constraints on heart transplantation today, only a small minority of patients warrant referral for transplantation. The consulting cardiologist should, however, understand the indications and contraindications for transplantation sufficiently well to recognize appropriate

candidates and to discourage exaggerated expectations from unrealistic patients (discussed in Chapter 17). Documentation of functional status may be as simple as recording the patient's New York Heart Association (NYHA) functional class in a chart note or as complex as performing formal maximal oxygen uptake testing. The critical clinical issue rests on ensuring that the degree of functional impairment corresponds to the severity of heart disease as assessed by other parameters. When disparity between the functional assessment and the anatomic or hemodynamic state exists, further investigation is required.

Finally, the cardiologist should provide regular monitoring consistent with the natural history of the patient's disease and access to tertiary-level health care, including clinical trials, parenteral therapy, surgery, electrophysiologic studies, and transplantation. As a consultant with a vast array of expensive and hazardous procedures to choose from, the cardiologist must serve as an advocate and interface between the patient and the technology of modern health care.

PRIMARY CARE ISSUES IN HEART FAILURE CARE

The primary care physician usually has the best perspective to offer an overview of a patient's health, particularly when viewed as an assessment of the effect of a disease process like heart failure on an individual's work, family life, and role in the community.

A critical question for many patients is, "Can I go back to work?" Answering the question requires an assessment of the physical and emotional demands of the job, a careful look at safety issues and knowledge of relevant industry regulations, discussion with industrial medicine personnel, if involved, evaluation of the patient's functional capacity, evaluation of arrhythmia and the potential for sudden death, and a realistic assessment of the social consequences of not returning to gainful employment.

Often, the primary care physician has useful knowledge about working conditions from other patients in the same plant, from community contacts, or other sources to which a consultant does not have ready access. On the other hand, a consultant who specializes in heart failure care may have a better sense of an individual patient's prognosis or a more realistic sense of a patient's functional capacity than does a nonspecialist. These unique perspectives should be shared before returning a patient to a job he or she should not be doing and before advising disability retirement for a patient still capable of enjoying the dignity and independence of earning a living.

In the context of the family, critical primary care issues involve identifying the patient's caregiver and evaluating his or her fitness for the tasks. Single patients, those whose spouse has a significant, limiting illness, and those with incomplete comprehension tend to have frequent readmissions for hospital care, consuming more resources than do other patients. The caregiver should attend educational and counseling sessions and actively participate in outpatient visits. The primary care visit should include an interim history and a summation session involving both the patient and the caregiver. In addition, patients need some private time with the physician to address sensitive issues; often this can best be done during the physical examination by allowing the patient some privacy and encouragement.

Primary care physicians often have a sense of the patient's role in the community. A respected teacher or business person who cannot meet the requirements of a full-time job may retain self-respect and avoid reactive depression by participating in church or volunteer organization activities. Often volunteering at the community hospital minimizes the inconvenience of frequent follow-ups while keeping patients active and interested in life. Primary care physicians can offer effective suggestions and encouragement for appropriate activity if they examine the opportunities available to their patients.

A number of well-conducted clinical investigations now support the contention that rehabilitation and exercise programs can improve functional capacity and quality of life for heart failure patients. The primary care physician can facilitate a referral to a quality rehabilitation program and offer encouragement to the patient who may be reluctant to undertake activity.

Finally, the primary care physician dealing with ambulatory heart failure patients should address a variety of noncardiac issues in this population, including the following.

1. *Appropriate health maintenance and screening.* Flexible sigmoidoscopy, rectal examination, mammography, Pap

smears and pelvic examinations, glaucoma screening, influenza and pneumonia immunization, and so on remain relevant to good long-term care for NYHA class I and II patients. In view of the dismal prognosis for patients with advanced heart failure, the arguments for extensive screening in that group become tenuous.

2. *Initiation of advance directives.* The patient and his or her family should be informed about the possibility of sudden and unexpected death in heart failure. Whenever possible, an advance directive, designation of a health care surrogate with limited power of attorney, and documentation of discussion should be in the primary physician's records, and the patient and the community hospital should have copies.

3. *Management of situational or reactive depression.* Heart failure patients may experience significant depression as they deal with substantial limitation of activity, recurrent hospitalizations, expensive and complex medication programs, and hemodynamically compromising arrhythmias. The primary care physician must recognize the emotional issues involved and deal with them in a straightforward, supportive manner. Fortunately, many patients respond well to the selective serotonin reuptake inhibitors now widely available for pharmacotherapy of depression, and cardiac side effects from these drugs are unusual.

The primary care physician has an important role in the care of the patient with chronic disease. In contrast to the technical issues confronting the cardiologist, the primary care physician must assist his or her patient in dealing with progressive loss of functional capacity and its consequences for the patient, the family, and the community.

SUGGESTED READING

De Marco T, Goldman L. Predicting outcomes in severe heart failure. Circulation 1997;95:2597–2599.

Nash IS, Nash DB, Fuster V. Do cardiologists do it better? J Am Coll Cardiol 1997;29:475–478.

Stevenson LW. Heart transplant centers: no longer the end of the road for heart failure. J Am Coll Cardiol 1996;27:1198–1200.

The Role of the Advanced Registered Nurse Practitioner in Heart Failure

Margaret Kay Worley

An advanced registered nurse practitioner (ARNP) is a registered nurse who has completed a formal course of study beyond the basic nursing education that has prepared him or her for specialized and advanced nursing practice in an expanded role. The nurse practitioner position was first developed in 1965 as a demonstration project based in community health to expand the nurse's role in well child care (1). Graduate-level course work now includes pharmacology, interpretation of laboratory findings, obtaining a health history, advanced physical and biopsychosocial assessment, physiology and pathophysiology of selected diseases and illnesses, and management and modification of selected therapies (2). An ARNP develops, through study and supervised clinical practice at the graduate level, expertise in a specific clinical area. This allows an ARNP to provide comprehensive care for patients with acute and chronic health needs within that area.

Currently, there are approximately 24,000 nurse practitioners practicing in the United States in a variety of settings (3). The Board of Nursing in most states defines the scope of practice for the nurse practitioner. Alaska and New Mexico permit an ARNP to practice independently from physicians, and 34 states have enacted statutes that allow an ARNP to practice without supervision as long as controlled substances are not prescribed. In the remaining states, an ARNP is required to have physician collaboration or physician supervision.

Specific parameters of collaborative practice are jointly established by the ARNP and the physician or group of physicians and are determined by the role or the description of practice within a particular setting and current legislative guidelines (4). An ARNP can function in both inpatient and outpatient settings. To provide services in the hospital, formal recognition of the ARNP as a patient care provider is necessary. This is achieved through the credentialing process and granting of clinical privileges. The Joint Commission on Accreditation of Healthcare Organizations allows the profession to "provide patient services in the granting institution, within well defined limits, based upon an individual's license and his/her experience, competence, ability and judgement." All individuals with clinical privileges are "subject to medical staff bylaws, rules, regulations and policies, and are subject to review as part of the hospital's quality assessment and improvement program" (5).

Nurse practitioners demonstrate a high level of autonomy and expert skills in diagnosis and management of patients with complex problems. Components of an ARNP's role include obtaining the medical history, conducting advanced physical exams, performing therapeutic interventions, coordinating patient care based on laboratory and diagnostic test results, adjusting medications and treatment plans, collaborating with other health care professionals in providing patient care, and providing education to the patient and family (6).

Heart failure patients have specialized needs that can be addressed efficiently and cost effectively when managed by a nurse practitioner in a collaborative practice. A collaborative practice is built in an atmosphere of mutual respect, trust, and commitment to quality patient care. This enhances the productivity of each practitioner by maximizing his or her expertise (7). This provides the framework for an increased efficiency and quality of care, decreased fragmentation of care, and overall satisfaction between the physician and the ARNP involved in the collaborative practice.

A sample of a collaborative practice protocol is shown in Figure 11.1. It is based on a practice that sees cardiology patients as both inpatients and outpatients in an academic setting. The practice protocol is an agreement between the ARNP and the physician and defines the scope of practice for the ARNP. It also outlines the degree of autonomy and supervision that is required for that practice. The sample protocol is consistent with the requirements set forth by the Florida State Board of Nursing.

Practice Protocol

I. Between

[Nurse Practitioner]
[Address]
[License Number]

and

[Physician]
[Address]
[License Number]

II. Nature of Practice

This collaborative agreement is to establish a practice that shall deliver adult cardiology care, including assessment, diagnosis, and treatment of cardiovascular disease, and health education and counseling. The practice shall be limited to clients in the [Name of group] both as outpatients at the [Office/clinic name and address] and on the inpatient services at [Name of hospital and address].

III. Duties of ARNP

Within the scope of this practice the ARNP shall be responsible for the following:

a. Perform initial history and physical examinations, both on an inpatient and outpatient basis, and identify medical problems.

b. Perform periodic physical examinations on inpatients.

c. Order appropriate laboratory tests, including x-rays, ECGs, echocardiograms, and exercise tests.

d. Draw blood specimens for testing and performing other comparable procedures when personnel who customarily perform such procedures are not available.

e. Order medications as defined in Section V.

f. Initiate consultations and monitor scheduling of patients for special tests.

g. Make daily rounds to observe and record pertinent progress of patients, updating and summarizing charts, and notifying responsible physician(s) of changes in patients' conditions.

h. Make interim summaries as required.

i. Dictate required notes on all procedures of preventive care, medical problems, and the use of prescriptive treatment and drugs, with the exception of the operative record.

j. Counsel the patient and his or her family about the preventive care, medical problems, and the use of prescribed treatments and drugs.

k. Start intravenous solutions and administer intravenous medications.

l. Manipulate and discontinue pulmonary artery catheters and peripheral arterial lines.

m. Perform clinical or research treadmills, bike or arm exercise testing on appropriate patients as per written protocols.

Figure 11.1: Sample patient protocol.

IV. Duties of Physician

The physician shall provide general supervision for routine health care and management of adult cardiovascular disease and provide consultation and/or accept referrals for complex health problems. Methods of supervision include, but are not limited to, case presentation and review. The physician or his or her designee shall be available by telephone or by electronic beeper when not physically available on premises.

V. Specific Management Areas

The conditions for which the ARNP may initiate and manage include, but are not limited to, angina, congestive heart failure, palpitations, chest pain, nicotine addition, hypercholesterolemia, and hypertension.

a. The following measures may be initiated by the ARNP:

Dietary prescription and counseling.
Activity prescription and counseling, including rehabilitation referral.
Wellness intervention.
Endocarditis prophylaxis.

b. When a patient for whom the ARNP is providing care is in a life-threatening situation, and when there is no licensed physician available, the following procedures may be performed:

(1) Manage cardiac arrest patients, including the use of external cardiac compression.
(2) Manage acute respiratory failure.
(3) Initiate cardiac defibrillation or cardioversion.
(4) Pass endotracheal tubes.
(5) Order and administer oxygen.
(6) Administer emergency medication per Advanced Cardiac Life Support (ACLS) guidelines.

c. The following types of medications may be initiated and/or renewed by the ARNP:

Analgesics
Anticoagulants
Antihistamines
Antacids
Anti-inflammatory agents
Antibacterials
Antihypertensives
Antianxiety agents
Bronchodilators
Cardiovascular agents
Contraceptives
Dermatologic agents
Diabetic agents
Diuretics
Electrolyte supplements
Emergency drugs
H2 antagonists
Hypolipidemic agents
Laxatives
Muscle relaxants
Ophthalmic solutions
Steroids
Vitamins and supplements

Figure 11.1: *(continued)*

d. Other measures may be initiated, depending on client condition and judgment of the ARNP.

e. All of the above functions may be performed under general supervision.

VI. Review of Agreement

Both parties to this agreement share equally in the responsibility for reviewing treatment protocols as needed and no less than annually.

[Signature]   [Signature]
_____   _____
[Typed ARNP name]   [Typed M.D. name]
[License Number]   [License Number]
Date:_____   Date:_____

Initiated: [Date]
Reviewed: [Date]

Figure 11.1:   (*continued*)

Reimbursement by third-party payer for ARNP-provided care varies. In many states, an ARNP may receive no direct reimbursement for the same services for which a physician may receive full payment. In other states, an ARNP may receive direct reimbursement but at a lesser rate than a physician for the same patient care services (8). This may influence the type of practice an ARNP may have with his or her physician collaborator.

ARNP CARE IN HEART FAILURE

An ARNP can play a central role in fostering independence and self-reliance in heart failure patients and the patients' families. An ARNP can provide intense patient education and reinforcement as well as serve as a primary contact point.

One area in which patients must receive ongoing education is on monitoring their weights daily and following a flexible diuretic schedule. Once they are on adequate doses of angiotensin-converting enzyme (ACE) inhibitors and digitalis, many patients require diuretics only when there is clinical evidence of fluid retention (9). Loop diuretics, including furosemide, bumetanide, torsemide, are the most commonly used and are among the most potent. The onset of diuresis in this group of drugs occurs within 1 h after administration, and the peak effect occurs within 2 h. If the patient returns to bed for 1 or 2 h after the morning dose, the diuretic effect may be enhanced (10). Because diuresis may last 6 to 8 h, patients on twice daily dosing should be encouraged to take the second dose in the late afternoon to avoid affecting the quality of rest at night. Some patients require the intermittent use of a second diuretic, such as metolazone, to augment the effect of the loop diuretic when a persistent weight gain occurs. Patients need clear-cut guidelines for when to take the supplemental medication, along with information about hypokalemia, hypotension, and dehydration (11–13).

Patients become more in tune to their heart failure symptoms and better comply with their drug regimens when they are given detailed written instructions, based on their individual weight, about how to adjust their specific diuretic therapy and how to restrict fluids and salt (Fig. 11.2). Patients also need specific information about when to call the office for worsening heart failure symptoms. Whether those symptoms include persistent weight gain, peripheral edema, orthopnea, increasing exercise intolerance, increasing abdominal girth, or early satiety. Once patients are taught the early clinical symptoms of heart failure, emergency room visits and hospital admissions may be avoided, because diuretic dose and nonpharmacologic therapy can be adjusted.

A second opportunity for patient education by the ARNP is in the area of anticoagulation management. Although there have been no randomized clinical trials on the use of anticoagulation therapy in patients with heart failure, these patients are considered at risk for thromboembolic disease because of their low cardiac output states, atrial and ventricular dilatation, and the increased incidence of atrial fibrillation (14). Most clinicians agree that low-intensity anticoagulation in this patient population is appropriate.

The most commonly prescribed oral anticoagulant is crystalline sodium warfarin. Warfarin prevents thrombosis by inducing a vitamin K deficiency. Low-intensity oral anticoagulation therapy with warfarin is initiated at 2 to 5 mg/day, and the prothrombin time–international normalized ratio (PT/INR) is measured on the day 3. When initiating therapy, serial monitoring of the PT/INR every 3 to 7 days is advised until the dose is stable, after which monitoring may be decreased to every 2 to 3 weeks and then every month. When adjusting doses, increase or decrease them by 10 to 20%, as

CHF Patient Instructions

Patient Name _____ MR# _____ Date _____

1. Weigh yourself every day and write it down! Weigh every morning after you have emptied your bladder. Your dry weight should be _____ pounds. Adjust your diuretic (water pill) if you gain more than 3–4 pounds over 2 days *or* you develop swelling in your feet/ankles. Call the office if your weight does not go down the next day.
2. You shouldn't drink more than _____ cc of fluid a day. This is the same as _____ ounces a day, or _____ cups. This includes coffee in the morning, tea, soda, juice, water with your medicines, *everything!* Keep track of exactly how much you drink each day. If you get thirsty, try sucking on hard candy (sugar free).
3. Do not eat more than 2 g (2000 mg) of sodium (salt) each day. Read the labels of food carefully to see how much salt is in each serving. Try to avoid processed foods, sandwich meat, pork, etc. *Do not* use a salt shaker when cooking. Try using other salt-free spices, fresh herbs, or lemon or lime juice.
4. Exercise some every day! Start out slowly, and gradually increase how much you do. *Do not* plan an activity for immediately after a meal or during the heat of the day. Remember that with your heart failure you can't do two activities at the same time, such as digest a meal and take a walk! Try to do something every day. On days that you feel good do more, on days you don't feel as well, do less.
5. Plan rest periods every day! Rest for 30–60 minutes after each meal.
6. Take your medications according to the following schedule:

Time	Activity/Medication	Description
6:00 A.M.	Get up	
	Weigh yourself*	
	Lasix 40 mg	Water pill
	Vasotec 20 mg	Reduces pressure load on the heart
	Digoxin 0.125 mg	Strengthens pumping of heart
	Lopressor 25 mg	Slows heart rate
	Go back to bed for 1 to 1½ hours	
7:30 A.M.	Breakfast	
9:00 A.M.	Go for a walk	
12:00 P.M.	Lunch	
	Rest	
4:00 P.M.	Lasix 20 mg	
6:00 P.M.	Vasotec 20 mg	
	Digoxin 0.125 mg	
	Coumadin 2.5 mg	Blood thinner
	Dinner	
	Rest	
9:00 P.M.	Plan light activity	
10:00 P.M.	Go to bed	

* If your weight is up take [water pill] today.

7. Check blood pressure daily and record. It is expected that your blood pressure will be between _____ and _____. Call the office if your blood pressure is less than _____ and you feel weak or dizzy when you stand up.
8. You will need to have your bleeding time checked on a regular basis (once a month) because you are on Coumadin. Your INR should be between _____ and _____.
9. Call _____, ARNP if you have any questions.

Figure 11.2: Sample CHF patient instructions.

appropriate, and monitor the PT/INR every 7 days to determine the dose adjustment needed (15).

The INR is a calculated PT ratio that takes into account local differences in prothrombin time reagents and equipment. Low-intensity anticoagulation is defined as an INR from 2 to 3; high-intensity anticoagulation is an INR of 3 to 4.5. Because the INR corrects for the variability in PT values obtained in different laboratories, its use allows for the best dosage decision for each patient (16).

There are several important considerations for the ARNP when initiating warfarin therapy. The first includes reviewing the patient's current list of medications to identify potential drug–drug interactions. In particular, amiodarone increases the anticoagulant effect of warfarin (17). Adding new medications to the patient's heart failure regime may mean monitoring the INR more frequently to ensure adequate anticoagulation and reduce the risks of bleeding.

Second, it is important to instruct the patient to avoid foods high in vitamin K. Foods that are high in vitamin K include Brussels sprouts, turnip greens, chickpeas, cauliflower, kale, spinach, beef and pork liver, and broccoli. Foods that are moderately high in vitamin K are coffee, rolled oats, cabbage, lettuce, asparagus, and Cheddar cheese (18). Other issues to discuss with patients are abstinence from alcohol and the use of an electric razor and a soft toothbrush. The ARNP should also stress the importance of regular monitoring. Patients must also remind other health care providers that they are on warfarin, because it should be stopped 3 to 4 days before any invasive procedure.

The third, and relatively new, area of opportunity for an ARNP in managing the patient with heart failure is with home infusion therapy. The goal of this therapy is to improve the patients' functional status and minimize hospitalizations in patients who are refractory to optimal medical treatment (19). An ARNP can determine if the patient is a candidate for home infusion therapy. Such patients are unresponsive to conventional therapy and thus require multiple admissions to the hospital for the management of congestive heart failure. Other candidates may include those not eligible for cardiac surgery or those awaiting surgery, including cardiac transplantation (20). Additional factors that need to be considered before home inotropic infusion therapy is started are patient's family support and the availability of experienced home health nurses and a clinical pharmacist. Finally, an adequate source of reimbursement should be a serious consideration in the decision-making process (21).

Home inotropic therapy requires that a patient have some type of central venous access device, either one with an implanted port, a peripherally inserted catheter, or a tunneled central chest catheter. The patient or family members will need to learn how to change dressings using a sterile technique, flush the catheter to maintain patency, and assess the insertion site for infection. An ARNP can initiate this education before the catheter is inserted and provide follow-up with the home health nurse.

No standardized optimal inotropic dosing regimen has been identified. The infusion times range from 4 to 72 h, and the frequency ranges from daily to once every 6 weeks (22). To minimize interruptions of daily life, 4 h twice a week has been effective in my patient population. The initial dose is the lowest effective dose, and up titration occurs as needed based on symptoms and response. During routine clinic visits with the ARNP, the patient can be assessed for efficacy of treatment, adverse effects of drug, laboratory monitoring, and need for additional therapy. An ARNP can also facilitate care with the home health nurse and the clinical pharmacist.

SUMMARY

The patient with heart failure presents a challenge to the health care provider. An ARNP, in addition to being clinically skilled, safe, and cost-effective, can provide high-quality care to this complex patient group.

REFERENCES
1. Ford LL. A deviant comes of age. Heart Lung 1997;26(2):87–91.
2. Board of Nursing. Rules of the Department of Professional Regulation. In: Administrative polices pertaining to certification of advanced registered nurse practitioners. Tallahassee, FL: Florida Board of Nursing, 1988:15–18.
3. Henry PF. Analysis of the nurse practitioner's legal relationships. Nurs Pract Forum 1996;7(6):5–6.
4. Knaus VL, Felten S, Burton S, et al. The use of nurse practitioners in the acute care setting. J Nurs Adm 1997;27(2):20–27.
5. The Joint Commission. Accreditation manuals for hospitals, vol. 1: Standards. Oakbrook Terrace, IL: Joint Commission on Accreditation of Healthcare Organizations, 1994.
6. American Association of Critical Care Nurses, American Nurses Association. Scope of clinical practice and scope of practice for the acute care nurse practitioner. Washington, DC: American Nurses, 1995.

7. Nugent KE, Lambert VA. The advance practice nurse in collaborative practice. Nurs Conn 1996;9(1):5–16.
8. Blouin AS, Brent NJ. Collide or collaborate? Changing reimbursement and legal challenges facing ANP and MD's. J Nurs Adm 1996;26(4):10–12.
9. Stevenson LW. Therapy tailored for symptomatic heart failure. Heart Fail 1995;11(3):87–107.
10. Mills RM. Management of the patient awaiting cardiac transplantation. Clin Cardiol 1992;15 (Suppl I):I28–I36.
11. Stevenson LW. Tailored therapy before transplantation for treatment of advanced heart failure: effective use of vasodilators and diuretics. J Heart Lung Transplant 1991;10(3):468–476.
12. Carson P. Pharmacologic treatment of congestive heart failure. Clin Cardiol 1996;19:271–277.
13. Baker DW, Konstam MA, Bottorff M, Pitt B. Management of heart failure: pharmacologic treatment. JAMA 1994;272(17):1361–1366.
14. Baker DW, Wright RF. Management of heart failure: anticoagulation for patients with heart failure due to left ventricular systolic dysfunction. JAMA 1994;272(20):1614–1618.
15. Fenstermacher K, Hudson BT. Practice guidelines for the family nurse practitioner. Philadelphia: WB Saunders, 1997.
16. Oertel LB. International normalize ratio (INR): an improved way to monitor oral anticoagulant therapy. Nurse Pract 1995;20(9):15–16, 21–22.
17. O'Reilly RA, Trager WF, Rettie AE, Goulart DA. Interaction of amiodarone with racemic warfarin and its separated enantiomorphs in humans. Clin Pharmacol Ther 1987;42:290–294.
18. Meluch F, Mitchell SB. Decreasing intracoronary stent complications. Dimens Crit Care Nurs 1997;16(3):114–121.
19. Miller LW. Outpatient dobutamine for refractory congestive heart failure: advantages, techniques and results. J Heart Lung Transplant 1991;10(3):482–487.
20. Mayes J, Carter C, Adams JE. Inotropic therapy in the home care setting: criteria, management, and implications. J Intraven Nurs 1995;18(6):301–306.
21. Coffin MR. Dobutamine infusion for the treatment of congestive heart failure in the home care setting. J Intraven Nurs 1994;17(3):145–150.
22. Berkland D. Creative solutions: home dobutamine infusions. AACN Clin Issues 1995;6(3):443–451.

Chapter 12

Ancillary Providers and the Care of the Heart Failure Patient

Roger M. Mills Jr.

The heart failure syndrome affects the individual patient, his or her family, and the entire fabric of that individual's network of social connection. A single physician, no matter how dedicated and skillful, cannot meet the myriad physical, psychosocial, and educational needs of the patient and the family. In today's health care system, the physician must call on a variety of ancillary providers to help with the six basic patient questions that are listed in Table 12.1.

This chapter examines the roles of a number of ancillary providers in the team-based care of the heart failure patient. The list is not all-inclusive but is intended to guide and to stimulate greater reliance on members of the team other than the physician. The roles are divided into those who primarily help the patient, those who help the physician, and those who help both patient and physician.

ANCILLARY PROVIDERS WHO HELP THE PATIENT

What Can I Do?

Physical therapy, home health services, and specialists in cardiopulmonary rehabilitation can help restore independence and function to patients debilitated or incapacitated by heart failure. Progressive activity in the hospital under supervision helps the patient gain confidence and strength. Often bed rest or limited activity helps restore cardiac compensation at the cost of orthostatic hypotension. The physical therapist should teach patients to sit before standing

Table 12.1.   The Six Questions All Patients Want to Ask

Question	Issues for the Answer
What can I do?	Guidelines for work, recreation, and sexual activity
What can I eat?	Salt and water limitations; dietary management of hyperlipidemia and diabetes
What medication do I take?	Formulary management, cost, effectiveness, compliance
Whom do I call when I have problems?	ARNP, primary, or specialty care; availability and responsiveness
How will I pay for all this?	Social issues; insurance versus government programs
What is going to happen to me?	Emotional issues; prognosis; anxiety and depression

ARNP, advanced registered nurse practitioner

and to use calf flexion to augment venous return instead of having the physician decrease the doses of angiotensin-converting enzyme (ACE) inhibitors.

The physical therapist assigned to work with heart failure patients in the hospital or in an outpatient setting must be aware of the diminished exercise tolerance and the degree of tachycardia often seen in heart failure and must set attainable goals for each patient. Stairs may be a huge obstacle for some patients, and patients should be encouraged to practice going up and down steps.

Outpatient rehabilitation programs not only build confidence but provide an opportunity for patients to share information and to function as part of a mutual support group. Learning that others have similar problems and sharing coping strategies can benefit patients as much as the physical rehabilitation process. Chapter 9 discusses the benefits of rehabilitation in detail.

What Should I Eat?

Dietary prescription and adherence to dietary restrictions are critical to the successful management of heart failure. Formal teaching for both the patient and the caregiver who buys, prepares, and serves the meals should include careful attention to appropriate caloric intake and dietary composition, including fat, sodium and potassium, fiber, and fluids. Whenever possible, a dietitian who has worked regularly with the heart failure team and who understands the approach to these issues should meet with the patient and his or her family. It is truly discouraging to see patients referred for heart transplantation *before* they are referred for dietary counseling and management.

ANCILLARY PROVIDERS WHO HELP THE PHYSICIAN

What Medications Do I Take?

Formulary management, drug interactions, and possible side effects complicate the polypharmacy to which most heart failure patients are subjected. The need for a program based on at least three or four drugs—including ACE inhibitors, digitalis, diuretics, nitrates, and often antiarrhythmics and anticoagulants; supplemental potassium and magnesium; and other drugs for comorbid conditions, such as diabetes or degenerative joint disease—raises endless questions about medications. Are the drugs chosen cost-effective, suitable for a convenient dosing schedule, and approved by the formulary under which the patient is covered? What potential drug–drug interactions may occur? What side effects must the patient be warned about, and how can this warning be documented? What dosing schedule should the patient follow? A clinical pharmacist oriented to the heart failure team can address all these questions and many others.

The heart failure team in my institution includes a pharmacist who joins rounds, reviews medication orders, and participates actively in discharge teaching for patients and families. Often, the clinical pharmacist will uncover critical issues, such as use of over-the-counter nonsteroidal anti-inflammatory drugs (NSAIDs) or prescriptions from other physicians that come to light only with repeated questioning.

Whom Do I Call When I Have Problems?

Chapter 11 addresses in detail the role of the advanced registered nurse practitioner (ARNP) in the care of the heart failure patient. A patient with a chronic progressive disease, such as heart failure, must know when his or her next scheduled medical visit will be and what to do if symptoms worsen or questions arise before that visit. A nurse or nurse practitioner trained in heart failure management can provide both urgent and scheduled continuing care for most patients, allowing the treating physician to focus on patients who have extremely complex problems or decompensated symptoms.

ANCILLARY PROVIDERS WHO HELP BOTH THE PATIENT AND THE PHYSICIAN

How Will I Pay for All This?

Chapter 13 reviews in detail the social issues involved in heart failure care. Patients need skilled social work intervention on several predictable occasions: at the onset of symptoms, when the question of disability arises, when recurrent episodes of decompensation raise the questions of noncompliance and inadequate resources at home, and when terminal or hospice care becomes appropriate. At each of these stages in the natural history of the disease, access to social resources and assessment of family, home care, and emotional support require more time and effort than a busy physician, concentrating on the physical and technical issues of patient care, can muster. The clinical social worker on the heart failure team can organize disability claims, recruit home health care providers, and help families deal with the progressive loss of function involved in heart failure. By addressing these issues, the social worker can prevent recurrent admissions and help maintain quality of life for many patients who would otherwise be caught in a revolving door pattern of hospitalizations.

What Is Going to Happen to Me?

Patients with heart disease uniformly experience depression and anxiety that, although often appropriate to their situation, frustrate their physicians. Acknowledging these emotional issues as valid and important allows the physician to open a discussion with the patient and family. Patients need to know that heart failure poses a serious threat to life and that the risk of sudden death is real and significant. The need for estate planning, advance directives concerning care, and the designation of an individual with health care power of attorney must be addressed. In this discussion, pointing out the emotional impact of the subject and offering an opportunity to work with a clinical psychologist to deal with these complex emotions indicates a physician's willingness to help with comprehensive care. Most patients and families respond well to simple, supportive interventions. For those with more complex issues, it may be critical to document that patient and family have been informed of the risks inherent to the heart failure syndrome.

Clinical and health psychology consultation, with continuing individual or family counseling, or referral to an appropriate support group will often improve compliance, reduce the attack-the-messenger hostility directed toward caregivers, and foster effective communication.

Finally, the treating physician should inquire about patient interest in pastoral care visits. Objective data confirm better outcomes in individuals with strong religious coping behaviors. No matter what mechanisms are involved, the pragmatic nature of medical care and a commitment to comprehensive care demand that the services be offered and used whenever possible.

SUMMARY

Caring for patients with a chronic, progressive, and ultimately fatal illness entails unique challenges. Effective use of resources, including the physician's time, energy, and emotional stores, demands a team approach to care. In such an environment, the physician serves as a manager, setting the tone, the goals, and the strategies of care, then calling on other members of the team to help with the myriad issues outlined above. This approach, employed effectively, can improve quality of life for patients and families. It calls on physicians to develop new habits of listening receptively to ancillary providers, building consensus among team members to support mutual goals, and of critically examining the evidence supporting medical decisions.

SUGGESTED READING

Allan R, Scheidt S. Heart and mind: the practice of cardiac psychology. Washington, DC: American Psychological Association, 1997.

American Society of Health-System Pharmacists. ASHP therapeutic guidelines on angiotensin-converting-enzyme inhibitors in patients with left ventricular dysfunction. Am J Health Syst Pharm 1997;54:299–313.

Braith RW, Mills RM Jr. Exercise training in patients with congestive heart failure. Postgrad Med 1994;96:119–130.

Kostis JB, Rosen RC, Cosgrove NM, et al. Nonpharmacologic therapy improves functional and emotional status in congestive heart failure. Chest 1994;106:996–1001.

Silver MA. Patient knowledge of fundamentals in chronic heart failure. Congest Heart Failure 1996;2:11–13.

Chapter 13

Social and Psychological Issues of Heart Failure

Roger M. Mills Jr. and Sharen Thompson

When we speak of heart failure, we may be referring to any of a variety of cardiac conditions, including coronary artery disease, atherosclerosis, cardiomyopathy, myocardial infarction, and congestive heart failure. However, regardless of the seriousness of the condition, life for patients and their families will change forever. In fact, the cognition itself that the patient is not the only one affected by a chronic cardiac condition can influence the nature of the response. Although characteristically diverse, cardiac conditions have in common similar psychosocial responses (1). Whether the patient experienced ventricular dysrhythmias without loss of consciousness or a full arrest with resuscitation, reactions by patients and families tend to fall into several identifiable categories: anger and depression, anxiety and emotional distress, denial with consequent lack of recommended lifestyle changes, cardiac cripples, and introspection with health-promoting lifestyle changes.

In almost all cases a patient's response to the diagnosis of heart disease may be affected by his or her physician's comments or reactions. In other words, patients who perceive that their doctors do not seem to be particularly worried about their heart disease may tend to minimize its seriousness and be less likely to see the need for any lifestyle changes. Physicians who smoke may weakly comment on the effect of cigarettes on the heart and de-emphasize the importance of smoking cessation. The same goes for doctors who are overweight. It is hard to present a convincing argument for change when physicians present themselves as such poor examples. In general, credibility (and perhaps compliance) increases when what is preached is also practiced.

TYPICAL RESPONSE

It is important first to examine typical responses and behaviors to chronic cardiac illness before defining strategies to cope with and eventually manage them. Reactions to heart failure vary, depending on personalities and on whether the heart failure developed slowly with reasonable compensation or if the onset was sudden, as in the case of acute failure. Reactions are also affected by the presence, responses, and support of the patient's family, employers, and other support sources, regardless of the composition of family involved.

Generally, patients and family members experience anger and depression, often as a result of feeling a lack of control over their lives. They may simply deny that there is anything wrong with them. They may continue smoking, drinking alcohol, eating unhealthy foods, or refuse to participate in a recommended exercise program.

For instance, Frank was 50 years old when his heart disease had progressed to the point at which a heart transplant was required. A construction supervisor at the same hospital where he underwent his transplant, Frank tried to monitor his crew from the hall window outside his hospital room. To his credit, Frank did return to work not long after his transplant. However, he continued to smoke cigarettes and engage in his evening ritual of watching television and eating a large bowl of chocolate and peanut candies.

Other patients may become cardiac cripples. They may quit their jobs, insist on being waited on, or withdraw from usual activities or social events.

One such case involved Travis, who had an emergent coronary artery bypass graft (CABG) directly following his first myocardial infarction (MI) at the age of 60. At just 5 years away from retiring, Travis seemed to be holding life in the palm of his hand. When it became evident that Travis would need to modify his demanding work schedule, he became severely depressed. For 6 months, Travis remained totally dependent on his wife, who unbegrudgingly attended to her husband's every need. She coaxed, coddled, and sometimes bribed him into getting out of bed in the morning. Recognizing the importance of mental stimulation, she would engage Travis in marathon sessions of board games and cards and the solving of jigsaw puzzles. Reflecting back on that time, she describes Travis as "requiring 24-h-a-day care."

For some patients, the shock of being diagnosed with heart disease may lead to introspection and lifestyle changes that are health promoting.

Sol was in his late 30s when he had a significant MI. Wondering why, at such a young age, this should happen to him, Sol elected to exercise some control over his life by modifying his diet, quitting cigarettes, and learning to identify stressful events as well as expanding his coping repertoire to include more positive responses to stress. Sol was medically managed successfully until the age of 70 when he underwent a five-vessel CABG. Acting on a life-long dream, Sol celebrated his 72nd birthday by taking a white water rafting trip down the Colorado River with his son and grandson.

It seems to be human nature to feel as though we would live forever. Our vulnerability can be dramatically realized when one is brought into a hospital, perhaps to have the heart shocked back into its life-sustaining rhythm or to have medications administered intravenously to augment the heart's functioning and help restore normal breathing. For individuals like Sol, it took one such event. For others, it may take many trips to the hospital before the precariousness of life is fully realized.

THE PSYCHOSOCIAL IMPACT OF CHRONIC CARDIAC DISEASE

Do not look back in anger, or forward in fear; but around in awareness.

James Thurber

Cardiovascular disease has long been the leading cause of mortality in the United States. With advancements in medicine, however, cardiovascular disease is now also the leading cause of morbidity. More people are living longer with chronic cardiac conditions. Studies abound on the subject of the emotional impact of cardiovascular disease, particularly in regard to its effect on the patient. However, the more comprehensive perspective of the whole person, or the psychosocial aspects of chronic cardiac disease, has just begun to be studied. It is also noteworthy that most of the research on individuals with cardiovascular disease has focused on men, leaving us less informed about women's adjustment to chronic cardiac illness. Questions are emerging regarding the effect of cardiovascular disease on women, its timely and appropriate diagnosing, and the development and implementation of effective treatment interventions.

Numerous studies have looked at the emotional impact of cardiac illness. The presence of depression, anxiety, anger, hostility, and emotional distress in patients with cardiac disease is well documented, although not necessarily well understood. For example, anxiety and depression can contribute to changes in eating and sleeping habits, which may be deleterious to one's health. However, the subsequent decline in one's medical condition can justifiably be attributed to a decline in cardiac functioning, and little attention is paid to the contribution of underlying anxiety or depression. More often than not, depression in patients with chronic cardiac conditions goes undiagnosed. When recognized, depression may be considered a normal concomitant of heart disease that requires no special attention or treatment.

Many studies have shown a positive relationship between inadequately treated depression and an increased rate of MIs and even death. Thus it would behoove physicians and patients alike to increase their awareness of various emotions associated with chronic cardiac illness.

Depression, as defined in the third edition, revised, of the *Diagnostic and Statistical Manual* (DSM–III-R), is marked by several characteristics, including but not limited to *(a)* a loss of interest and pleasure, which can extend to family, friends, and activities; *(b)* appetite disturbance, which usually presents as a decrease in appetite but may manifest as increased consumption; *(c)* sleep disturbance, which can be experienced as either insomnia or its opposite, hypersomnia; *(d)* psychomotor disturbance, which may be experienced as a decrease in energy level; and *(e)* an overall decreased sense of self-worth, which may be accompanied by reduced joy in life. These may all be psychological and behavioral indicators of depression, which can easily contribute to and be attributed to cardiovascular disease.

Anger can be a useful emotion when used constructively, such as for considering alternatives and problem resolution. Left to fester, anger can wreak havoc physically, resulting in increased blood pressure, muscle tension, and a weakening of the body's immune system. Studies of chronically hostile people show that they have increased blood pressure accompanied by higher levels of adrenaline and cortisol in their blood compared to nonhostile individuals. Hostile people also tend to engage in such health-compromising behaviors as smoking, substance abuse, and overeating (2). People who are emotionally distressed tend to have more frequent doctor visits for such somatic complaints as dizziness, headaches, fatigue, and pain and are more often hospitalized than are less-stressed individuals. Consequently, emotional distress itself often goes unrecognized. Left untreated, the true needs of the patient remain unresolved, which can lead to ineffective care and frustration for both the patient and physician.

DEPRESSION

My surgeon understood the symptoms, but only I know the underlying cause.

Richard Bode

There are numerous reasons why individuals with chronic cardiac illness may become depressed, angry, anxious, distressed, or hostile. Experiencing a brush with death can contribute to feelings of intense vulnerability. Patients may begin to think about all they stand to lose or all they would miss if they were to die. A certain amount of life review takes place, at which time patients may begin to challenge their accomplishments, raise regrets, or question such existential issues as the meaning of their lives. Some patients may worry about losing their jobs or going on disability, with its reduction in finances. Others may embrace the opportunity to stop working but may question their ability to actively participate in life and enjoy such pleasures as dancing, fishing, traveling, gardening, and sex. Still others may ruminate about their spouse and minor children, wondering who will care and provide for them. When cardiac disease significantly impinges on one's source of personal satisfaction and gratification, a sharp decrease in subjective well-being may be predicted (3).

Faced with a life-threatening and often disabling illness, a questionable sense of personal competence, marital role changes, family disruption, financial strains, reductions in social activity, emotional stress, and the shattering of many hopes and dreams, chronic heart failure patients are understandably anxious, depressed, or angry. Advances in medicine have made chronic cardiac illness a reality for more and more people. The struggle becomes not only one of staying alive but also one of figuring out how to add quality, meaning, and purpose to life.

CHRONIC CARDIAC DISEASE—A FAMILY AFFAIR

Out of clutter, find simplicity. From discord, find harmony. In the middle of difficulty lies opportunity.

Albert Einstein

Wayne was 44 years old when he was diagnosed with end-stage cardiac disease. Married with young children, Wayne struggled to work as long as possible. When he finally did agree to stop working and apply for disability income, his application was denied. For 2 years Wayne fought his case, which eventually went to court; the judge ruled in Wayne's favor. During those 2 years, however, Wayne's life was turned upside down. Always able to provide for his family, Wayne's wife now had to secure a job. Although she was able to obtain a part-time, minimum-wage position, she had not worked since her late teens and lacked the skills for substantial employment. With money tight, the family was constantly in jeopardy of losing its home or having the utilities turned off. Wayne had considerable difficulty adjusting to the imposed lifestyle changes. Not only was he unable to work but he was limited in what he could do around the house and with his children. Before long, Wayne became severely depressed. His children began having problems both in and out of school. Wayne's wife thought often about "running away" as the stress became too much for her.

The Neglected Family

At the initial diagnosis and then with each subsequent exacerbation, concentrated attention is paid largely to the patient. People do not, however, live in a vacuum. An acute or chronic cardiac condition has a ripple effect that touches, and often changes, the lives of many people. Spouses may neglect their own health care needs. The role of disciplinarian may be assumed by the spouse. Extreme efforts may be taken to maintain peace within the home so as not to upset the patient and possibly cause a heart attack. Older adolescents may need to take a job after school to augment the family's income. Plans to go away to college may be canceled. The straight-A student may see his or her grades slip. Younger children may need to assume more household responsibilities. Older children may be needed to care for younger children. Adult children who have been independent may need to move back in with a parent. Plans to start a family may be put on hold or canceled altogether if a patient becomes too ill. Death may need to be confronted sooner than anticipated. What helps the spouse, the children, the patient, or the family unit survive and possibly even thrive during this time?

Support

Many patients and family members make reference to the support they receive from others as being helpful and healing. What, though, is meant by *support?* Social support can be defined as the psychosocial and tangible aid provided by a social network (family, friends, others) and received by a person (4). Emotional support includes the expression, either verbal or behavioral, of caring, concern, and acceptance. Feelings and actions are affirmed through active listening and the expressed understanding of another's feelings. Emotional support conveys a sense of being there for the patient, the spouse, the children, or others as needed. Support can also be informational, through, for example, the sharing of knowledge, the exploration of options, and the development of strategies to enhance coping and encourage problem solving. Tangible aid can include identifying resources and providing assistance with household tasks and help with daily activities.

The type of social support considered beneficial varies among patients and family members. Emotional support may be more important for family members during a crisis event, such as an episode requiring hospitalization, life-threatening arrhythmias, or sudden death. As the crisis component subsides, family members may have a greater need for informational or tangible aid. Once stable, patients may require emotional support yet may not be ready to receive information or benefit from direct tangible aid. Informational support may be more important during the time when patients are actively adjusting to changes in roles and lifestyle (5).

For example, at 8:00 P.M., the on-call social worker was asked to go to the medical intensive care unit to provide support to Tom's immediate family members. Tom, at age 36, was diagnosed with inoperable heart disease. He was not a candidate for bypass surgery or transplantation. It seemed evident that Tom would not survive the night. Present were his wife, 14-year-old daughter, and 10-year-old son. Tom's wife and daughter chose to spend the night in the hospital. His son opted to leave and spend the night with his coach. Conversations with Tom's daughter revealed her sadness about her father missing her high school graduation in the years to come. She was also able to express her disappointment that he would not be there to walk her down the aisle on her wedding day. Tom's daughter was actively, and appropriately, grieving. Tom's wife, was able to both accept counseling from available staff and provide support to her daughter. Tom's son needed time to understand and accept his father's illness and eventual demise. Fortunately, his coach was responsive and empathic. Tom's son was able to share many of his concerns, fears, and sadness with his coach, which he could not do with his immediate family or hospital staff. Tom's wife expressed concern regarding her children's adjustment to their father's death. She was interested in obtaining information about local bereavement groups, counseling, bibliotherapy, peer support, and anything else that might help her children cope with the loss of their father. She readily accepted support from friends who brought over dinners, co-workers who covered her position at work, and church members who helped with the children.

Support must be viewed as a dynamic process that is tailored to meet the individual's needs as much as possible. The type of support helpful to a patient's 10-year-old daughter is different from that needed by the patient's 76-year-old father. What a newly diagnosed patient needs will differ from someone who has lived with cardiac disease for many years. What would be helpful to a spouse with four young children is likely to be very different from that of a single person with no children.

Support for patients and family members should not be limited to an acute or crisis event. Emotional, informational, and tangible support ideally should be available to patients and family members alike throughout the course of a chronic illness. Support need not solely come from a spouse or one companion or only health care professionals. Extended family, friends, support groups, and even pets can provide support that is accepted by the individual as beneficial.

LIVING WITH CHRONIC CARDIOVASCULAR DISEASE

Chronic cardiac disease is *forever:* lifelong for the patient, lifelong for the family. With time, everyone adjusts. Typical stages of adjustment include initial shock and disbelief, followed by periods of apprehension and exhilaration. On one hand, patients may become apprehensive about never quite feeling safe with their compromised heart, while at other times they may feel exhilarated simply to be alive. Family members, too, experience shock, disbelief, apprehension, and exhilaration, although not necessarily in the same order or at the same time as the patient or as one another. Just as it takes time for a patient to adjust and return to a new normal lifestyle, family members also need time to heal and recover (6).

Family members are not static. As individuals within the family mature, their needs and behaviors may change. For minor children, it is helpful to inform key personnel at school so that they can be cognizant of subtle changes in grades or behavior. As children grow into adolescents, a previously devoted and involved child may become more distant. The opposite can also occur; children who seemed distant and unconcerned may in their teen years spend more time at home and may cling to the ill parent. The spouse is also maturing. Periodic feelings of disappointment, resentment, confusion, and exhaustion are normal. It is essential for spouses, on a routine basis, to monitor their physical and emotional health. Spouses who use a supportive network of friends and family generally cope better than do spouses who are isolated or overburdened with responsibility and have limited or constructive outlets.

STRATEGIES

Life is lumpy. A lump in the oatmeal, a lump in the throat, and a lump in a breast are not the same lump. Problem or inconvenience? One should learn the difference.

Robert Fulghum

Few of us appreciate what we have until we lose it. Catching a cold can be an inconvenience. Having life-threatening arrhythmias is a problem. It seems natural to focus on what we do not have rather than on what we do have and to perceive all losses as problems. On some days, living with chronic cardiovascular disease is an inconvenience. On other days, it is very much a problem. Either way, the chronic cardiac condition remains. It does not go away. Yet some days are better than others. The challenge of living with chronic cardiovascular disease is to try to maximize the periods of inconvenience and reduce the problem times. Easy to say, yet hard to do . . . or is it?

There are some known strategies that are positively associated with reducing the risk or possibly retarding the advancement of cardiovascular disease. They include changes in diet, smoking, exercise, sexual activity, and stress management. Most strategies are more successfully implemented when all family members are actively involved rather than just the patient.

Diet

A change in dietary habits is an example of a strategy that can have a positive effect on the heart patient's health. Studies have shown that young children and their parents share similar levels of cardiovascular risk characteristics (7). High serum cholesterol levels and obesity are traits that tend to run in families. The link between cholesterol and heart disease is strongest in young and middle-aged males. This is the group most at risk of premature heart disease and death. Obesity can contribute to high blood pressure, diabetes, and stroke. Therefore, it seems that all family members would stand to benefit from changing their eating habits.

There is no conclusive evidence that extreme changes in diet will guarantee a longer, healthier life. However, dietary modifications, particularly if started early, cannot hurt and may prove beneficial. Basic dietary modifications include such steps as adding generous amounts of foods rich in soluble fiber and eliminating many processed foods that contain saturated fats, such as palm and coconut oil. Salt has been noted to have a deleterious effect, particularly on patients diagnosed with high blood pressure. Eliminating or significantly restricting salt consumption often aids blood pressure regulation. Again, there is strength in numbers; if all other family members continue the salt habit, the odds are great that the patient will too.

Adjustments made together have the most staying power. Eating habits are more likely to be successfully changed when foods rich in flavor and texture are part of each meal. Fortunately, the market abounds with cookbooks containing recipes designed to be health promoting while maintaining the integrity and good taste of food. Changing one's eating habits may be frustrating and inconvenient in the short run but may reduce the risk of serious cardiovascular problems in the long run.

Smoking

Perhaps the most difficult habit to change is cigarette smoking. The American College of Physicians' Health and Public Policy Committee found that 90% of smokers would like to quit and about 15% actually attempt to stop their habit each year. Two-thirds of those who are able to quit do so entirely on their own. Many patients express concern that since they have smoked for so long, there may be no real value to quitting. The Framingham Study looked at 26,000 people and found that within 5 to 10 years of quitting, the risk of a smoker experiencing a future heart attack decreases to that of a nonsmoker (8). While there is good documentation about the positive effects of quitting, many people still have difficulty achieving long-term abstinence. Enlisting the support of family members can be helpful. If patient and spouse both smoke, their commitment to stopping may be greater if they stop together, giving each other reinforcement.

Smoking is both physically and psychologically addicting. A good smoking cessation program, therefore, must address both problems. Many programs exist; they can be categorized into five major techniques: *(a)* drug therapy, *(b)* behavior modification, *(c)* educational and commercial programs, *(d)* hypnosis, and *(e)* multiple risk factor reduction. If a particular program does not work for a particular patient, another program should be tried. Each program offers something different. Patients who express a desire to quit on their own should be encouraged to do so while also being informed about the existence of programs for future reference. Smoking is a problem. Smoking cessation is difficult but not impossible. Continued cigarette use will increase the risk of cardiovascular events and associated complications.

Ron continued to smoke long after he was advised by several physicians to quit. After becoming a chronic cardiac patient who subsequently developed diabetes, Ron still refused to quit smoking. Eventually, Ron underwent several amputations to his lower and upper extremities. Until the day he died, Ron smoked cigarettes.

Exercise and Cardiac Rehabilitation

The positive relationship between exercise and cardiovascular disease has been well documented. Some well-known benefits of exercise include lowering blood pressure; raising blood volume, which reduces stress on the heart; increasing HDL levels; obviating depression; and suppressing the appetite, which helps control weight and improves cardiac efficiency.

Following a cardiac event, patients and family members are often filled with feelings of uncertainty, ambivalence, and confusion about which activities can be safely done and which should be avoided. Participation in a formal cardiac rehabilitation program may serve to mollify anxiety, since patients physical functioning is professionally monitored. In addition, information regarding their disease is provided, and patients are educated about cardiovascular risk factors and appropriate health-promoting behaviors. Ideally, spouses should be included in as many of the sessions as possible to reduce the possibility of differences over medical instructions.

One reason patients give for not participating in cardiac rehabilitation is inconvenience. Most would agree, however, that it is not nearly as inconvenient as having a major cardiac event, which can result in a hospital admission and possible death. The dominant goal of cardiac rehabilitation is to assist patients in achieving an optimum quality of life (9). Teaching and counseling are offered to help patients regain their previous or optimum level of physical, vocational, and social activities. In addition to the aforementioned benefits of physical exercise, cardiac rehabilitation may increase the likelihood that a patient who is deemed medically able to work actually does so.

A study that looked at the return to work rate of patients with acute myocardial infarctions found no difference among patients who did and those who did not participate in a formal cardiac rehabilitation program (10). However, long-term studies that looked at patients 2 and 5 years later, found significant increases in the rate of return to work among the patients who did undergo cardiac rehabilitation. This was particularly true in men less than 55 years old.

Patients who are exposed to a formal occupational or vocational evaluation tend to resume employment more quickly than those who receive no such intervention. Clearly, the potential problems to patients, families, and society, resulting from reduced return to work rates far exceed the inconvenience of participating in a formal cardiac rehabilitation program.

Sexual Activity

Another common concern of patients and families that can affect quality of life is the resumption of sexual activity. Anxiety and fear associated with a cardiac event often leads to reduced sexual activity or sexual dysfunction (11). Most patients and spouses would like to know more about how their cardiac condition affects their sexual activity. The tendency, however, is for patients to receive less information about sexual activity than about such matters as exercise, smoking, diet, and returning to work. The discrepancy between the information provided and the information desired may be a result of the discomfort patients, spouses, and physicians tend to experience when discussing sexual matters openly. Many cardiac rehabilitation programs offer sexual counseling, which may be effective in assisting patients and spouses with resuming a comfortable level of sexual activity.

For example, Art was 64 years old when he experienced a significant cardiovascular event, which resulted in an emergent evaluation for possible cardiac transplantation. Mary, his wife, was in her late 50s. When questioned about their sexual activity, Mary reported that the couple had not been sexually active for 10 years. Approximately 2 months following Art's transplant, Mary called to say that Art was interested in resuming their sexual relationship. Mary, however, was not. With counseling, the couple decided not to resume coitus, but they are physically close with one another. Periodically, Art teases Mary about "finding a sweet young mistress," to which Mary responds by offering to help her husband pack his bags and show him out the front door. This couple has successfully negotiated their differences regarding their sexual relationship. They engage in an active lifestyle and enjoy one another's company immensely.

Stress Management

The emotional component of cardiovascular disease warrants addressing, particularly in light of the positive relationship found between negative emotions and an increased risk of cardiovascular disease. Fortunately, many techniques exist that are designed to help individuals manage stress, defuse negative emotions, and develop a coping repertoire composed of healthy alternatives.

Numerous strategies exist for managing stress. Some simple examples are socializing with friends, watching a favorite movie, listening to music, reading a good book, or taking a nap. Others may take more coordination or planning, such as playing a team sport, doing volunteer work, taking a long walk, or taking a long warm bath. Meditation and keeping a personal journal are also effective stress reducers. Stress often is a matter of perception. A change in one's perception can dramatically reduce the experience of stress. Differentiating between something being a problem or an inconvenience may be all that is needed.

> For instance, Jon was in his early 30s and recently married when his cardiomyopathy was first diagnosed. At that time he headed a lucrative landscaping business, which he was reluctant to give up. As Jon's health deteriorated, his physician more assertively argued for Jon to change careers. Though initially very upset, Jon soon realized that giving up the landscaping business would enable him to go back to school and eventually pursue his lifelong desire to be a teacher. Careful consideration of all that it meant to give up his business turned what at first appeared to be a significant problem into a minor inconvenience. Jon now receives disability benefits as well as assistance with his education expenses through the Department of Vocational Rehabilitation. Jon and his wife quickly learned to adjust to the changes in their financial situation. In spite of decreased finances and increased health problems, Jon acknowledges being a much happier person.

Negative emotions can be successfully diffused by recognizing that one can choose the manner in which they respond to anger, frustration, and disappointment. The need to feel in control is essential to many chronic cardiac patients. Yet, they can all too easily explode when angry and then apologize by saying, "I couldn't help myself." Patients can help themselves and can maintain control by recognizing that there is more than one way to respond to an incident.

Helping patients and family members to expand their coping repertoire can result in more effective and appropriate responses to difficult situations, while also helping them to recognize and manage stressful events. Additional coping strategies include the use of cognitive thought stopping, which employs cognitive analysis of a thought to challenge irrational beliefs and fears coupled with the exchange of a negative thought for a positive thought. Temporary distraction and withdrawal can help one to cool off. The appropriate use of humor and laughter can help diffuse a potentially explosive situation, while having a healing effect on the body by expelling carbon dioxide, increasing the intake of oxygen, relaxing muscles, and lowering heart rate and blood pressure. Taking several slow, deep breaths can also slow the pulse and relax muscles.

Volunteering or participating in organized groups can serve to fight feelings of isolation and expand one's capacity for empathy. A heart-to-heart talk with a close friend or calling a minister, priest, or rabbi can be beneficial.

SUMMARY

Although the physical manifestations of heart failure vary, the effect on patients and families remains consistent. Given the wealth of documentation regarding the positive correlation between cardiovascular disease, psychosocial adjustment, and improvement of quality of life, it is incumbent on health care providers to assume an holistic approach to patient care.

One last suggestion: Don't sweat the small stuff. Remember it is *all* small stuff.

REFERENCES

1. Kolar JA, Dracup K. Psychosocial adjustment of patients with ventricular dysrhythmias. J Cardiovasc Nurs 1990;4:44–55.
2. Sobel DS, Ornstein R. Defusing anger and hostility. Ment Med Update 1995;4:3–5.
3. Waltz M. Marital context and post-infarction quality of life: is it social support or something more? Soc Sci Med 1986;22:791–805.
4. Fleury J. An exploration of the role of social networks in cardiovascular risk reduction. Heart Lung 1993;22:134–144.
5. Yates BC, Skaggs BG, Parker JD. Theoretical perspectives on the nature of social support in cardiovascular illness. J Cardiovasc Nurs 1994;9:1–15.
6. Castelli J. I'm too young to have a heart attack. Rocklin, CA: Prima, 1990.
7. Deutscher S, Epstein FH, Kjelsberg M. Familiar aggregation of factors associated with coronary heart disease. Circulation 1966;33:911.
8. Cohn PF, Cohn JK. Heart Talk. Cambridge, MA: Harcourt Brace Jovanovich, 1987.
9. Froelicher ES, Kee LL, Newton KM, et al. Return to work, sexual activity, and other activities after acute myocardial infarction. Heart Lung 1994;23:423–435.
10. Hedback B, Perk J. Five-year results of a comprehensive rehabilitation programme after myocardial infarction. Eur Heart J 1987;8:234–242.
11. Mann S, Yates JE, Raftery EB. The effects of myocardial infarction on sexual activity. J Cardiac Rehab 1981;1:187–192.

Chapter 14

What Constitutes Quality in the Management of Heart Failure?

Eileen Handberg and Roger M. Mills Jr.

Heart failure (HF), as outlined in the previous chapters, is a complex syndrome with a variety of causes. Development can be acute or chronic; and as a result, patients present along a continuum from asymptomatic with left ventricular dysfunction to symptomatic with overt heart failure and pulmonary edema. Because of the multifactorial nature of the symptoms, treatment options also become multifaceted. Interventions may be focused on correction of the underlying cause (i.e., revascularization for ischemic heart disease) and/or alleviation or palliation of symptoms (i.e., shortness of breath owing to volume overload).

With all of the therapeutic options available and the wealth of ongoing research, how do health-care providers ensure that HF patients receive quality care? Should quality be measured based on improvements in symptoms, changes in morbidity and mortality, or economic outcomes? With the current focus on health care expenditures, the primary measure of quality patient management appears to be targeting the economic aspects of providing care. Many market factors influence the push toward quality care programs in health care. Increasingly, hospitals and health care systems compete for technology and patients, during a time of reduced health care dollars. As a result, health care systems are attempting to restructure services to develop better use of resources and reduction of costs, while maintaining quality health care. In these restructured services, new programs are often targeted to specific diseases or diagnoses, such as HF, which make up a significant portion of health care expenditures.

The staggering cost of HF helps explain the effort that has been expended on establishing quality programs to better manage patients. HF is a debilitating, fatal syndrome that affects 1 to 2% of the adult population; there are 400,000 new cases annually in the United States (1). HF incidence has continued to increase, despite reductions in acute and chronic coronary disease and stroke rates. HF management costs have been estimated at $10 billion annually to cover costs of hospitalizations, outpatient care, and medical therapy (2). In 1991, nonfederal hospitals reported 2,280,445 discharges with a primary or secondary HF code. The average length of stay was 7.7 days, including 3 days in the intensive care unit. These hospital admissions alone cost $5.45 billion, which accounted for 4.8% of the diagnosis-related group (DRG) budget (3). In 1992, Medicare paid $2.4 billion for 654,000 hospital admissions for HF. The actual charges were $5.6 billion, with a mean charge of $8500 (2). These costs reflect frequent hospitalizations for diagnosis and treatment, in addition to subsequent rehospitalizations to optimize therapy in decompensated patients.

Surveys of 90-day readmission rates for HF patients ranged from 19 to 42% (4,5). In a 3-year review of HF patient admissions at one southern California hospital, it was documented that financial losses averaged $2.5 million annually, in spite of reduced length of stay and above-average reimbursement rate. These losses were believed to be the result of a high rehospitalization rate, which is an indicator of inadequate maintenance and follow-up care of this chronically ill population (6). Clearly, even moderate changes in practice that result in reduced lengths of stay or readmission rates could have a significant effect.

Quality health care has been defined as "attained when the needs and expectations of the customer are met with a minimum of effort, rework and waste. . . . Patient outcomes are the goals of planned health-care interventions, developed as a measure of the quality standard care" (7). How do practitioners meet the needs of the patient and also benefit the health care delivery system through a standardized quality HF care program? Can they be complementary? Can a goal of providing quality care both improve patient outcomes and reduce health care expenditures? To implement a standardized quality program, it is important to understand the state of current HF management and to decide if changes in practice can meet these goals.

QUALITY MEASURES AND QUALITY ISSUES

In 1991, the Agency for Health Care Policy and Research (AHCPR) appointed a panel to develop HF practice guidelines. This panel, made up of experts in fields pertinent to HF and lay personnel, reviewed available research to determine which interventions could alter outcomes. They developed clinical practice guidelines based on the available scientific literature; published in 1994, the guidelines detail all aspects of HF management (2). The initial review of the literature identified several major trials that clearly demonstrated surgical or pharmacologic interventions that could reduce morbidity and mortality in this population. The panel then identified common errors in diagnosis, evaluation, testing, and management. Based on currently available information about optimal HF care, these errors reflect a lack of quality.

The management errors are listed in Table 14.1; errors such as these actually do result in adverse outcomes. Kosecoff et al. (8) found that 12% of patients hospitalized with HF received poor or very poor quality care as explicitly defined prospectively. Common errors included early discharge of unstable patients, which resulted in a 16% 90-day mortality rate compared to a 10% rate for stable patients.

The results of the Studies of Left Ventricular Dysfunction (SOLVD) Trial, a National Institutes of Health–sponsored placebo-controlled trial to evaluate the addition of the angiotensin-converting enzyme (ACE) inhibitor enalapril to standard therapy in patients with chronic symptomatic HF, was published in 1991 (9). The data from 2569 patients showed that ACE inhibitor therapy led to a 22% reduction in risk of recurrent heart failure and a 26% reduction in rehospitalization for worsening heart failure. A study of prescribing practices before and after the publication of the SOLVD report found that 24% of HF patients in 1990 were receiving ACE inhibitor therapy, but by 1992, the use of ACE inhibitors in HF patients had increased to only 31% (10).

This less than optimal therapy appears to be related to two factors: differences in practitioner prescription patterns and the demographics of who manages HF in the outpatient setting. The majority (83%) of HF patients are cared for by noncardiologist physicians; however, the majority of prescriptions for ACE inhibitors are written by cardi-

Table 14.1.   Errors in Management

- Coexistent hypertension is often not treated aggressively enough
- Patient, family, and caregiver education is often inadequate
- Patients with heart failure not due to systolic dysfunction may be treated inappropriately
- Practitioners may not instruct patients to monitor their weight closely
- Patient noncompliance and its causes are often not recognized and dealt with appropriately
- The possibility of revascularization is often not considered in patients who have severe coronary artery disease with left ventricular systolic dysfunction
- Patients with severe heart failure are often referred too late for heart transplantation, after severe decompensation and development of secondary multisystem organ failure
- Exercise prescriptions are underused
- Angiotensin-converting enzyme inhibitors are not initiated or are prescribed at suboptimal doses because of clinician's concerns about possible side effects
- Physicians frequently prescribe inadequate doses of diuretics in patients who continue to have overt volume overload despite modest doses of diuretics
- Practitioners may fail to appreciate the potentially deleterious effects of certain pharmacologic agents in heart failure (e.g., calcium blockers, nonsteroidal anti-inflammatory agents, β-agonist inhalers)

From Konstam MA, Dracup K, Baker DN, et al. Heart failure: evaluation and care of patients with left-ventricular systolic dysfunction [Clinical practice guideline No. 11; AHCPR publication 94-0612]. Rockville, MD: Agency for Health Care Policy and Research, June 1994.

ologists. It has been estimated that less than 20% of the initial prescriptions written by family practitioners and internists for patients with HF included ACE inhibitor therapy. It is alarming that lack of or inadequate administration of ACE inhibitors persisted 4 years after the SOLVD results were published. This failure to translate life-saving clinical research into clinical practice is one of many indications of quality problems in HF management.

The care of HF patients is increasing in technical complexity, and the volume of new data from clinical research is considerable. In some respects, practitioners have legitimate concerns about the translation of clinical research to practice. The AHCPR panel reviewed more than 1000 articles, of which 237 were used to develop the guidelines. The process required the panel to make decisions on the relative value of the research based on both subjective and objective data (11). An individual practitioner cannot assimilate all of the available literature and base his or her practice on scientific evidence in isolation. In fact, most physicians do not alter their prescribing habits significantly once they leave training. The demonstration that ACE inhibitors are grossly underprescribed raises concerns for the future. If the delay in translation from clinical research findings to clinical practice persists, quality care will suffer and the cost of care will continue to escalate.

CLINICAL PRACTICE GUIDELINES

If clinical research findings are not currently readily translated into practice, can practice guidelines help practitioners deal with the technical complexity of HF management? And what are practice guidelines?

Clinical practice guidelines are recommendations, based on the current scientific literature, to assist in determining how diseases, disorders, and health care conditions can most effectively and appropriately be prevented, diagnosed, treated, and managed clinically (2). Guidelines are usually developed by professional and/or regulatory groups made up of experts in the field. They are designed to be a concise document to guide practice. Practicing physicians have sometimes viewed guidelines with suspicion. Guidelines have been decried as cookbook medicine that ignores the clinician's judgment. Others have expressed concerns that guidelines will be used to dictate licensure or certification or to determine reimbursements.

More than 1400 guidelines have been or are currently being developed by at least 30 different commissions and 80 professional organizations (12). For heart failure, there are at least two major sets of recommendations: the AHCPR guidelines (2) and the American College of Cardiology/American Heart Association (ACC/AHA) guidelines (13). Both sets of guidelines were written by experts in the field of HF management. The AHCPR panel included a diverse group of practitioners (physicians, nurses, pharmacists) and consumer representatives; whereas the ACC/AHA Task Force was composed exclusively of physicians. The guidelines were disseminated through the scientific literature and other media to practicing physicians and other health care providers, including pharmacists and nurses, who help manage patients with HF (14,15). The AHCPR guidelines are also available in an abbreviated version that is targeted specifically to patients and families.

Once written and disseminated, how well are guidelines followed? In a review of compliance with practice guidelines, Grilli and Lomas (16) identified 143 medical recommendations with compliance data reported. The mean compliance rate was 54.5%; and compliance in cardiology was slightly higher (63.6%). Recommendations about highly complex procedures had lower reported compliance than those that were less complex (41.9 versus 55.9%). The target areas of practice, complexity, and trainability (the extent to which a procedure can be experimented with on a limited basis before making a final decision to adopt) appear to be partial useful predictors of the level of compliance with a practice guideline.

In one evaluation of compliance, Ellrodt et al. (17) measured physician compliance with a locally developed chest pain clinical practice guideline. They retrospectively reviewed an intervention trial designed to implement the practice guidelines to reduce length of hospital stay for low-risk patients with chest pain. The initial intervention of implementing guidelines was considered successful with a prestudy compliance rate of 50% and a poststudy compliance rate of 69%. This change in practice resulted in significant reduction in length of stay and a cost reduction of approximately $1397 per low-risk patient.

The analysis examined the actual activities of the guideline implementation. During the study period, 230 patients were classified as low-risk. Of those patients, 151 were discharged according to guidelines. The remaining 79 patients, who had hospital stays greater than 3 days, were initially classified as noncompliant. Of those correctly categorized as low-risk at admission, 9% required a change in classification owing to a change in clinical status and 14% were not discharged because of system inefficiencies (e.g., waiting for tests to be completed, for test results to be released, for nursing home placement). In 15%, the increase in stay had no identifiable reason, and 16% had an increased length of stay because their physicians refused to discharge them.

In summary, there are many reasons for noncompliance. Without careful review, a practitioner might be labeled as not cooperating with the guidelines. Ellrodt et al.'s in-depth review of the circumstances of each case indicated that clinical decision making for these patients was complicated. In fact, as independent researchers who reviewed all of the data, they agreed that 5 of the 13 patients should not have been discharged.

This study highlights several pertinent issues. Guidelines are useful tools for targeting changes in practice. Guidelines should "guide," not mandate, care and they cannot take the place of decision-making skills. Before charging a physician with noncompliance, a careful evaluation must be conducted to determine the exact cause. All aspects of guideline implementation should be evaluated fairly and should consider all issues, such as system delays and changes in clinical status, that may affect a physician's ability to comply with a guideline.

Targets for guidelines include both inpatient and outpatient management. In a recent European survey of current practice patterns for prevention of coronary heart disease in light of published recommendations (18), there was a significant gap between the cholesterol levels thought to confer increased risk requiring treatment and thresholds for actual treatment (with lipid-lowering drugs and/or diet). For patients with cholesterol levels between 6.5 and 8.0 mmol/L, there was a range of nontreatment of 8 to 45%. Clearly, there is a gap between dissemination and adoption of guidelines in many areas of cardiovascular disease.

LOCAL GUIDELINES: CRITICAL PATHS

Clinical practice guidelines offer a great potential service to health care providers, compiling a wealth of data into a concise document that can be used to guide practice. Figure 14.1 illustrates the AHCPR clinical algorithm for HF management. It consolidates a review of the scientific literature into a one-page, easy-to-follow diagram.

Certainly, individual implementation will positively affect the care of a practitioner's patients. The real benefit to society, however, is through the widespread adoption of these guidelines. For HF guidelines to be successful, practitioners must be aware of the guidelines, intellectually agree with them, adopt them, and then adhere to them. The emergence of managed care and capitation has forced institutions to examine their practice patterns and to improve the quality to reduce costs. At the level of local or integrated health care delivery, clinical practice guidelines are often adapted and per-

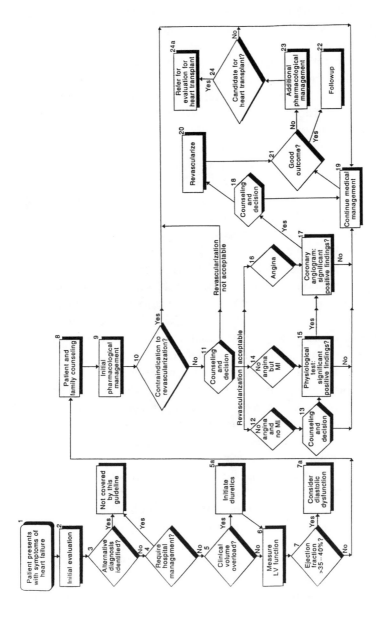

Figure 14.1: Clinical algorithm for evaluation and care of patients with heart failure. From Konstam MA, Dracup K, Baker DW, et al. Heart failure: evaluation and care of patients with left-ventricular systolic dysfunction [Clinical practice guideline No. 11; AHCPR publication 94-0612]. Rockville, MD: Agency for Health Care Policy and Research, June 1994.

sonalized to reflect the nuances of the implementing organization. The quality assurance literature is replete with articles documenting the development and implementation of quality-assurance programs for specific disease states, including HF (6,19,20). These are found as clinical practice guidelines, critical paths, care plans, or checklists.

For HF practice guidelines to be accepted locally, they must reflect both the most current scientific information available and the local environment. The environment includes not only physical resources (e.g., hospital beds, technology), personnel resources, (e.g., physicians, nurses, and other health care providers), and ancillary services (e.g., discharge planners) but also financial resources. The makeup of insurance carriers, health maintenance organizations (HMOs), and preferred provider organizations (PPOs) that pay for hospital services can greatly affect choices in implementation of guidelines.

The success of HF guideline implementation requires the buy-in of the local health care providers. Key among the factors that lead to this success is the inclusion of all parties in the planning stages of implementation. A team approach is necessary, especially in heart failure because of its multifactorial nature. A team might consist of a variety of providers such as family practitioners; internists; cardiologists; nursing services; social services; discharge planners; and department heads for areas of high technical service, such as the cardiac catheterization laboratory and echocardiography laboratory. Support personnel within the facility, such as dietitians and social workers, also need to be educated about streamlining services and accommodating changes. The team approach allows all areas to work together to ensure the best chance at being successful.

Once a team had been convened it is important to determine what the current patterns of care are within the institution. Extensive clinical data analysis is necessary to determine what is currently happening within the institution. Billing records must be carefully examined to determine the actual use of resources. Once the patterns of practice have been documented, variations must be identified and explored. Variations in areas such as charges, length of stay, intensive care unit stays, pharmacy charges, and use of ancillary services offer excellent starting places for designing and implementing interventions.

Education is an extremely important quality team function. All areas affected by the HF practice guidelines will need attention.

Physicians and other health care providers need to understand the rationale for guidelines and the expected outcomes that will result with implementation, specifically reductions in cost and the affect on patient outcome. The researchers who developed the chest pain guidelines (17) demonstrated that patient mortality and morbidity were not increased when low-risk patients were discharged within 2 days. Sharing this information with treating physicians presumably helped eliminate impediments to success by assuring practitioners that the changes in practice did not increase risk for their patients. Similarly, the AHCPR guidelines demonstrate that certain therapies reduce morbidity and mortality.

Before an institution embraces guidelines, a predefined evaluation process should be in place. The entire process is a dynamic one that will change over time as our knowledge of HF increases. Therapies will change and our evaluation of effectiveness may change. This evaluation should examine all areas of the guidelines program, from length of stay and costs of care to patient satisfaction.

At our institution, a tertiary referral facility in the U.S. Southeast, a team composed of practitioners (physicians and nurses) and department heads developed a critical path to standardize care of HF patients (Fig. 14.2). The AHCPR clinical algorithm (Fig. 14.1) can also be used as a framework for a local structure. Fairly complete examples of clinical path development at other institutions are also available (2,6,13,19,21).

As noted above, heart failure requires both inpatient and outpatient management. While changes in inpatient care can significantly reduce cost, optimization of outpatient care may have the greatest effect on total health care expenditures through an ultimate reduction in hospital admissions. As indicated previously, lack of consistent maintenance care and outpatient follow-up account for the high 30- and 90-day hospital readmission rates. Development of clinical pathways should not end with the discharge of the patient but must also incorporate comprehensive outpatient management strategies.

Several models of comprehensive outpatient management strategies to reduce rehospitalizations are available. Aggressive management of HF patients in nurse or nurse practitioner clinics can reduce rehospitalization rates, significantly affecting health care expenditures for HF (20,22). The difficulty with outpatient management programs in the private sector is the education and coordination of

SHANDS

at the University of Florida

The Clinical Pathway is a general guideline. Patient care continues to require individualization based on patient needs and requirements.

CLINICAL PATHWAY
TITLE: HEART FAILURE [Exclusion: I A B P]
SERVICE: CARDIOLOGY

Patient Name: MR#:

ALLERGY ALERT: •Note all allergies and check to ensure patient receives no medication allergic to. Call service to obtain alternative medications.
Shaded area = MICU only

CARE ELEMENT	Admission Day 1 Date:	Day 2 Date:
CARE UNIT	Cath Lab MICU 54 IMC	MICU 54 IMC
CONSULTS	•Nutrition •Social Services	————————————→ •Social Services •Consult with PT to evaluate re cardiac rehab
TESTS/LABS Notify HO for: PTT <40 or >100	•RDB, CBC, LFT,PT/INR if on Coumadin •PTT q 6 hr, if anticoagulated until PTT >60 x 2 •CXR PA & lat on admission per order •12 lead EKG on admission per order	•RDB in AM •PTT if heparinized
ASSESSMENTS Notify MD •SBP < 80 > 140 •HR < 60 > 120 •RR > 30 •O² sat <90% •VT, > 10 PVCs per min, frequent multifocal PVCs •PCWP <15 or >25 mHg •CI <2.5 •SVR <800 or >1200	•VS q 15 min when titrating meds; then q hr •PCWP & PAD initially; if wedge within 1-2 of PAD, don't wedge - readings q 4hrs •Assess effects of inotropes q 4 hrs •Systems assessment qs •I & O qs •Weight on admission •Monitor rhythm	•Swan Ganz readings q 4 hrs •Assess effects of inotropes q 4 hrs •Systems assessment qs •I & O qs •Weight qd •Monitor rhythm
TREATMENTS	•IV ML or PICC - flush qs with NS •If applicable, Swan Ganz catheter (MICU) •Cardiac monitor •O2 at ____ LPM •O2 sat monitor •Titrate 0₂ to keep Sat >92% •Evaluate for DC O2 and Sat monitor once stable - may D/C O² & monitor if O² sat >92% on room air	•IV ML or PICC - flush qs with NS •If hemodynamic goal achieved, d/c Swan Ganz catheter (MICU) •Cardiac monitor •O2 at ____ LPM •O2 sat monitor •Titrate 0₂ to keep Sat >92% •Evaluate for DC O2 and sat monitor once stable- may D/C O² & monitor if O² sat >92% on room air

MEDICATION	•Electrolyte replacements per protocol
	•Titrate inotropes to keep SBP 85-110, PCWP 18-20, Woods
	 units <3.0, UO > 30 cc/hr
	•Meds per MD orders:
	   •ACE inhibitors
	   •Vasodilators
	   •Diuretics
	   •Digoxin
	   •Anticoagulant per order
		•Electrolyte replacements per MICU protocol
		•Titrate inotropes to keep SBP 85-110, PCWP 18-20, Woods
		 units <3.0, UO > 30 cc/hr
		•Meds per MD orders:
		   •ACE inhibitors
		   •Vasodilators
		   •Diuretics
		   •Digoxin
		   •Anticoagulant per order

PAIN/SYMPTOM CONTROL	•Tylenol 650 mg PO q 6 PRN pain or HA •Maalox TC 15 cc PO q 6 hr indigestion •MOM 30 cc PO q 8 hr constipation •Benadryl 25-50 mg PO q HS sleep •Xanax 0.125 mg PO q 8 hr anxiety	•Tylenol 650 mg PO q 6 PRN pain or HA •Maalox TC 15 cc PO q 6 hr indigestion •MOM 30 cc PO q 8 hr constipation •Benadryl 25-50 mg PO q HS sleep •Xanax 0.125 mg PO q 8 hr anxiety
ACTIVITY	•Bedrest while Swan Ganz in place or titrating inotropic drugs •BSC if stable •Assist w/ ADLs	•OOB to chair with assist & BSC if stable •Progress w/ADLs
NUTRITION	•CCU 2 gm Na, low fat, NCS FR 1500 cc	•CCU 2 gm Na, low fat, NCS •FR 1500 cc
DC PLANNING/ TEACHING	•Assess knowledge deficit re CHF •Explain monitors, tubes, lines •Explain purpose of meds & ionotropic support •Explain purpose of Na and fluid restriction, daily weights to patient/ significant other Assist Heart Transplant Coordinator w/pre-tx teaching (if indicated)	•Explain low Na, low fat diet, no caffeine or stimulants •Explain meds as they are converted from IV to PO •Reinforce purpose of daily wts, I & O, & fluid restriction •Teach about knowledge deficits of CHF and cardiac tx, if applicable

COPYRIGHT © 1996 SHANDS at the University of Florida

Figure 14.2: Critical pathway for inpatient management of heart failure patients. Reprinted with permission from SHANDS, University of Florida, Copyright 1996.

large groups of private practitioners. The effort will more than pay for itself, however, if patients can be aggressively managed. Many large health care systems and HMOs now use clinical pathways to standardize the outpatient care of HF patients. The goal is to monitor the patients closely and reduce exacerbations of failure. This requires targeting patients' and families' educational needs to foster indepen-

CARE ELEMENT	Day 3 Date:	Day 4 Date:	Day 5 Date:
CARE UNIT	•MICU •54 IMC	•54 IMC •54	•54
CONSULTS			
TESTS/LABS Notify IIO for: PTT <40 or >100	•RDB •PTT if heparinized •PT/INR if coumadin	•RDB •PTT if heparinized	•RDB •PTT if heparinized
ASSESSMENTS Notify MD •SBP < 80 > 140 •HR < 60 > 120 •RR > 30 •O² sat <90% •VT > 10 PVCs per min, frequent multifocal PVCs •PCWP <45 or >25 mHg •CI <25 elim 1m² •SVR <800 or >1200 dynes/sec/cm-5	•VS q 15 min when titrating meds; then q 1 hr •Assess effects of inotropes q 4 hrs •Systems assessment qs •I & O qs •Weight qd •Monitor rhythm	•VS q 2-4 after weaned from inotropic support •Systems assessment qs •I & O qs •Weight qd	•VS q 4 hr •Systems assessment qs •I & O qs •Weight qd
TREATMENTS	•IV ML or PICC - flush qs with NS •If hemodynamic goal achieved, d/c Swan Ganz catheter(MICU) •Cardiac monitor •O2 at ____ LPM - may D/C O² & monitor if O² sat >92% on room air	•IV ML PICC - flush qs with NS •DC Swan Ganz per MD •Cardiac Monitor •O2 at ____ LPM - may D/C O² & monitor if O² sat >92% on room air •DC foley cath, if applicable	•DC ML before d/c •Telemetry if ordered •D/C O² per MD order
MEDICATION	•Electrolytes as needed •Titrate/wean IV inotropic support •Meds per MD orders: •ACE inhibitors •Vasodilators •Diuretics •Digoxin •Anticoagulant per order	•PO meds •Wean IV inotropic support over 2-6 hrs •Meds per MD orders: •ACE inhibitors •Vasodilators •Diuretics •Digoxin •Anticoagulant per order	•ASA 1 po qd •PO meds •Meds per MD orders: •ACE inhibitors •Vasodilators •Diuretics •Digoxin •Anticoagulant per order
PAIN/SYMPTOM CONTROL	•Tylenol 650 mg PO q 6 PRN pain or HA •Maalox TC 15 cc PO q 6 hr indigestion •MOM 30 cc PO q 8 hr constipation •Benadryl 25-50 mg PO q HS sleep •Xanax 0.125 mg PO q 8 hr anxiety	•Tylenol 650 mg PO q 6 PRN pain or HA •Maalox TC 15 cc PO q 6 hr indigestion •MOM 30 cc PO q 8 hr constipation •Benadryl 25-50 mg PO q HS sleep •Xanax 0.125 mg PO q 8 hr anxiety	•Tylenol 650 mg PO q 6 PRN pain or HA •Maalox TC 15 cc PO q 8 hr indigestion •MOM 30 cc PO q 8 hr constipation •Benadryl 25-50 mg PO q HS sleep •Xanax 0.125 mg PO q 8 hr anxiety
ACTIVITY	•OOB to chair tid with meals and a.m. care •Ambulate w/assistance in room •Progress with ADLs	•OOB to chair with meals a.m. care •Ambulate in hallway as tolerated. •Progress with ADLs	•Resume usual activity level •Ambulate in hallway as tolerated. •Progress with ADLs
NUTRITION	•CCU 2 gm Na, low fat, NCS •FR 1500 cc	•CCU 2 gm Na, low fat, NCS •FR 1500 cc	•CCU 2 gm Na, low fat, NCS •FR 1500 cc
DC PLANNING/ TEACHING	•Reinforce diet instruction in low Na, low fat diet •Instruct patient to identify meds as they are given •Ask patient to explain purpose of I & O, wts and fluid restriction •Have patient monitor own fluid restriction •Teach S/S of worsening CHF: SOB, DOE, activity intolerance, increased HR, increased edema, decreased UOP, weight gain •Evaluate for homecare follow up; contact care manager or home care clinician	•Have patient list foods high in Na. •Have patient explain purpose of each med •Have patient identify each med •Teach patient major SE of each med •Have patient state S/S of worsening CHF •Reinforce principles of cardiac rehab per PT •Discuss home care need with case managers/home care liasion if indicated	•Ask patient to explain fluid and dietary restriction •Have patient state purpose and major SEs of each discharge med •Have patient list at least 5 S&S of worsening CHF •Have patient/ significant other verbalize plan for follow-up care

Figure 14.2: *(continued)*

dence and self-management, while providing adequate access to resources. These managed-care plans rely on ancillary services, such as social services, home health care, and hospice, to provide support. The ability to self-monitor HF creates a partnership between patient and provider that fosters success in outpatient management programs.

SUMMARY

O'Connell and Bristow (3) recommended the development of regional HF centers, similar to those developed for cancer research and treatment. These centers could provide a cohesive organizational structure for optimal HF therapy; and by working with local primary-care providers, patients could be maintained on optimal therapy with ready access to centers dedicated to state-of-the-art HF management. As health care providers, we want to provide the best chance for improved quality of life for patients with HF. Incorporating currently available clinical practice guidelines into local care pathways will go a long way toward achieving the goal of care based on the strength of well-conducted research.

Clearly, changes in the health care marketplace advocate quality assurance to reduce cost. In contrast, we argue for the adoption of practice guidelines to reduce morbidity, to eliminate recurrent heart failure, and to improve both the quality and quantity of remaining life for the heart failure patient.

REFERENCES
1. American Heart Association. Heart and stroke facts. Dallas: American Heart Association, 1995.
2. Konstam MA, Dracup K, Baker DW, et al. Heart failure: evaluation and care of patients with left-ventricular systolic dysfunction [Clinical practice guideline No. 11; AHCPR publication 94-0612]. Rockville, MD: Agency for Health Care Policy and Research, June 1994.
3. O'Connell JB, Bristow MR. Economic impact of heart failure in the United States: time for a different approach. J Heart Lung Transplant 1994;12:S107–112.
4. Cardiology Preeminence Roundtable. Beyond four walls. Research summary for clinicians and administrators on CHF management. Washington, DC: The Advisory Board Company, 1994.
5. Rich MW, Freedland KE. Effect of DRG's on three-month readmission rate of geriatric patients with congestive heart failure. Am J Public Health 1988;78: 680–682.
6. Brass-Mynderse, NJ. Disease management for chronic congestive heart failure. J Cardiovasc Nurs 1996;11(1):54–62.
7. Pare DS, Freed MD. Clinical practice guidelines for quality patient outcomes. Nurs Clin North Am 1995;30(2):183–196.

8. Kosecoff J, Kahn KL, Rogers WH, et al. Prospective payment system and the impairment at discharge: the "quicker and sicker" story revisited. JAMA 1990;264;1980–1983.
9. The SOLVD Investigators. Effect of enalapril on survival in patients with reduced left ventricular ejection fractions and congestive heart failure. N Engl J Med 1991;325:293–302.
10. Rajfer SI. Perspectives of the pharmaceutical industry on the development of new drugs for heart failure. J Am Coll Cardiol 1993;22(Suppl A);198A–200A.
11. Hadorn DC, Baker D, Hodges JS, Hicks N. Rating the quality of evidence for clinical practice guidelines. J Clin Epidemiol 1996;49(7):749–754.
12. Sandrick K. Out in front: managed care helps push clinical guidelines forward. Hospitals 1993;67:30.
13. Ritchie JL, Cheitlin MD, Eagle KA, et al. ACC/AHA Task Force report. Guidelines for the evaluation and management of heart failure. J Am Coll Cardiol 1995;26(5):1376–1398.
14. Anonymous. ACC/AHA collaborate on guidelines for the evaluation and management of heart failure [Editorial]. Am Fam Phys 1996;53(6):2196–2198.
15. Anonymous. Diagnostic and treatment mistakes add to costs of heart failure care [Editorial]. Am J Hosp Pharm 1994;51:2076.
16. Grilli R, Lomas J. Evaluating the message: the relationship between compliance rate and the subject of a practice guideline. Med Care 1994;32:202–213.
17. Ellrodt AG, Conner L, Riedinger M, Weingarten S. Measuring and improving physician compliance with clinical practice guidelines. Ann Intern Med 1995; 122:277–282.
18. Shepard J, Pratt M. Prevention of coronary heart disease in clinical practice; a commentary on current treatment patterns in six European countries in relation to published recommendations. Cardiology 1996;87:1–5.
19. Lauver LS. Benchmarking: improving outcomes for the congestive heart failure population. J Nurs Care Qual 1996;10(3):7–11.
20. Rich MW, Beckham V, Wittenberg C, et al. A multidisciplinary intervention to prevent the readmission of elderly patients with congestive heart failure. N Engl J Med 1995;333:1190–1195.
21. Welsh C, McCafferty M. Congestive heart failure: A continuum of care. J Nurs Care Qual 1996;24–32.
22. Kornowski R, Zeeli D, Averbuch M, et al. Intensive home-care surveillance prevents hospitalization and improves morbidity rates among elderly patients with severe congestive heart failure. Am Heart J 1995;129:762–766.

Chapter 15

Checklists for the Practicing Physician

Roger M. Mills Jr.

As a physician and a licensed pilot, I am fascinated by the numbers of physicians who have had at least some rudimentary aviation training and by the many similarities between doctoring and flying. Both require a careful blend of science for understanding, artful technique for smooth execution, good judgment, and occasionally a dash of pure luck.

On my first day as a student pilot, I met the preflight checklist; and I have never flown without verifying it. Checklists effectively organize repetitive tasks for which inattention, distraction, or failure to confirm a step can lead to problems, some of which are minor, some major, and some life-threatening. The clinician evaluating a new patient, discharging a patient after an episode of hospital care, or seeing the patient in routine follow-up faces similar problems: innumerable small issues, many distractions, and a situation that carries significant potential risk. Checklists provide an important safety mechanism when used properly, with the understanding that no one can remember all the steps all the time.

The three checklists presented in this chapter have been designed to cover the most common complex interactions between physicians and heart failure patients: initial evaluation, hospital discharge, and office follow-up. Each setting has unique aspects that favor the checklist approach. You may wish to customize the lists to fit your own needs. They offer a good place from which to start.

THE INITIAL EVALUATION CHECKLIST

The initial evaluation requires gathering enough clinical and laboratory data to accomplish several goals, including *(a)* making an accurate clinical diagnosis; *(b)* assessing the patient's current level of functional impairment; *(c)* assessing the psychosocial effect of the functional impairment, the potential for treatment, and the potential for rehabilitation; and *(d)* gathering the initial data required to "risk stratify" the patient in regard to appropriateness of various interventions.

Figure 15.1 presents a checklist for the initial evaluation. The personal history defines the patient's functional context in terms of family, friends, occupation, and major activities. Only by gathering this background information can the physician begin to understand the effect of the patient's cardiac limitations on the individual and his or her surroundings.

The detailed cardiac history explores the onset and evolution of the patient's cardiac disease. Whenever possible, obtain records from previous admissions and procedures to substantiate the patient's recollection. In this careful review, problems and issues often become much more clearly defined as relatively acute or chronic. The physician and patient together often gain a better understanding of the natural history of disease as manifested in a particular individual. The typically episodic and incremental deterioration of coronary disease often contrasts dramatically with the slow insidious decline seen with valvular or congenital disease.

As the discussion moves to other aspects of the medical history, the physician should carefully delineate other processes that may either mask or exaggerate cardiac symptoms. Conditions such as symptomatic peripheral vascular disease or major orthopedic problems may not only mask cardiac symptoms but also call into question the wisdom of attempting high-risk procedures that will have minimal effect on the patient's overall ability to perform physical activities. Similarly, symptomatic chronic pulmonary disease may substantially worsen the perception of dyspnea and may also dramatically increase the risk of surgical intervention.

Metabolic conditions such as exogenous obesity, uncontrolled hyperlipidemia, or chronic diabetes significantly limit the range of options available to any given individual. For example, when initially evaluating the heart failure patient, the clinical cardiologist should bear in mind the difficulty obtaining appropriate cardiac donations for patients weighing over 100 kg and the substantial adverse effect of diabetes on the postcardiac transplant course. The overall history

1. Personal History

Age
Sex
Reproductive status
Marital status
Occupation and employment status
Alcohol, tobacco, substance abuse habits
Military and/or travel history
Recreation (athletics, hobbies, recreation, and pursuits)
Family history

2. Detailed Cardiac History

Onset of clinical heart disease
Hospitalizations
Procedures, diagnostic
Procedures, therapeutic
Current therapy
Current symptoms
NYHA class

3. Other Medical History

Comorbidity
Metabolic status (diabetes, lipids, weight)

Objectives: A reasonable assessment of who this person is, what he or she does, how much difficulty is he or she encountering in daily life, and the current management program.

4. Physical Examination

Height	Weight	BMI
Resting pulse	BP	RR
Carotid bruits		
Neck veins		
Rales		
Apical impulse		
Parasternal lift		
Palpable gallop		
Paradoxical S_2		
Diastolic sounds		
Murmurs		
Liver pulsatile		
Femoral and distal pulses		
Edema		

Objectives: Assessment of volume status, both intravascular and extravascular; assessment of filling pressures hemodynamic status, ventricular function, and comorbidity

5. General Laboratory

- All patients:
  CBC
  Renal function, electrolytes
  Thyroid
  Blood type (If any consideration of transplant)
  Chest film/ECG
  Echocardiogram

Figure 15.1: A checklist for the initial evaluation of heart failure patients.

- Most patients:
  Pulmonary functions
  24–48-h Holter monitor

6. Special Studies

Diagnostic right and left heart catheterization
Electrophysiologic testing
Maximal cardiopulmonary exercise test
Right heart hemodynamics (on maintenance therapy)

Objectives: Complete anatomic diagnosis; detailed functional assessment of heart and lungs; risk assessment: functional, anatomic, electrophysiologic; plan of treatment

Figure 15.1:   (*continued*)

facilitates a reasonable assessment of who the person is, what he or she does, how much difficulty he or she is encountering in daily life, and what attempts to intervene have already been made.

The physical examination should routinely include a careful assessment of both height and weight and the calculation of body mass index (BMI). The BMI has become a widely accepted measure of obesity, and a measure greater than 30 kg/m² requires attention as a distinct medical problem under the heading of morbid obesity. These patients must be counseled that substantial weight loss will often markedly increase their functional capacity, and some may even be considered for bariatric surgical intervention.

In the cardiovascular evaluation of patients with symptomatic heart failure, a global assessment should dominate the physical examination. Individuals with resting tachycardia, cool hands and feet, and any impairment of mental status should generally be considered candidates for prompt hospitalization. Resting tachycardia in particular indicates perilously low stroke volume, high sympathetic tone, and the need for more vigorous medical interventions. A careful search for extravascular disease and an assessment of overall volume status are also critical to the initial evaluation. In the decompensated patient, auscultation of the heart is usually unrewarding. The rapid heart rate, prominent summation gallop, and functional murmurs of mitral and tricuspid regurgitation tend to obscure more subtle findings.

The objectives for the physical examination include a good assessment of intravascular and extravascular volume status, estimation of filling pressures in the pulmonary and systemic circulations, clinical assessment of hemodynamic status and ventricular function, and the effect of comorbidities.

The general laboratory evaluation includes a complete blood count (CBC) as part of the assessment of oxygen-carrying capacity, an evaluation of renal function and electrolyte status as part of the patient's overall fluid management, and a laboratory assessment of thyroid status. Even though uncommon, the profound effect of thyroid disease on cardiovascular function warrants laboratory assessment. Documentation of blood type should be obtained if there is any consideration of transplantation, since patients with type O blood now face considerably longer pretransplant waits than those with any other blood type. A chest x-ray, resting 12-lead electrocardiogram, and two-dimensional and Doppler echocardiogram complete the initial laboratory evaluation. The echocardiogram reveals such a wealth of anatomic and hemodynamic information that it has become an integral part of the clinical database in the assessment of these patients.

In addition, for most patients, a complete set of pulmonary function studies should be obtained once the individual has returned to hemodynamic compensation. In addition, if a recent period of continuous ECG monitoring is not available, 24 to 48 h of ambulatory electrocardiographic monitoring should be obtained in most heart failure patients, given the high incidence of sudden death in this population.

Special studies include diagnostic right and left heart catheterization to document coronary anatomy and hemodynamic status and electrophysiologic testing if significant arrhythmia has been detected by history, routine laboratory studies, or ambulatory monitoring. For risk assessment, a cardiopulmonary exercise test with measurement of maximum oxygen uptake ($\dot{V}O_2max$), right heart catheterization for assessment of pulmonary artery pressures, pulmonary vascular resistance, and right and left heart filling pressures should be obtained as part of the initial database. The objectives of the special laboratory studies include a complete and definitive anatomic diagnosis; a detailed assessment of both cardiac and pulmonary function; and a risk assessment based on anatomic, functional, and electrophysiologic data. These findings should allow a complete plan of treatment.

THE QUALITY INDICATOR CHECKLIST FOR HOSPITAL DISCHARGE

The hospital discharge checklist (Fig. 15.2) ensures that relevant diagnostic data have been gathered, therapy has been maximized, and ancillary support services personnel (who have a great deal to offer the heart failure patient) have participated in care. If all these steps have been covered, then the discharging physician and the patient will share the goals of preventing recurrent decompensation and avoiding readmission.

The anatomic diagnosis should be documented. The possible role of arrhythmia in precipitating symptoms, exacerbating the anatomic problems, or putting the patient at risk of sudden death should be considered and appropriate management steps confirmed. A recent assessment of ventricular function should be available for most patients, particularly if a marked change in clinical status has occurred.

1. Diagnostic

Anatomic diagnosis?
Arrhythmia management?
Ventricular function quantitation? (as clinically appropriate)
NYHA class?

2. Therapeutic

Scheduled times for medications?
Converting-enzyme inhibitor therapy at maximal doses?
Diuretic therapy minimized?
Dietary salt and water limitations?
Daily weight adjustments detailed?
Risk–benefit issues discussed, particularly in regard to anticoagulants, amiodarone?
Advance directive issues addressed?
Clinical trials considered?

3. Consultations

Clinical/health psychology
Dietitian
Financial counselor
Home health services
Pastoral care
Pharmacist
Physical therapy/rehabilitation
Social services

Figure 15.2:   A discharge quality indicators checklist.

Finally, the clinician should document New York Heart Association (NYHA) classification on admission and discharge, to clarify the patient's functional status after therapeutic intervention.

The discharge checklist requires the physician to spend a modest amount of time and effort reviewing precisely how the patient should manage his or her schedule at home. Having specific scheduled times for medication doses helps maintain therapeutic drug levels and avoids intermittent activation of neurohumoral responses, which should be continuously blocked.

Hospitalization should include an attempt to maximize angiotensin-converting enzyme (ACE) inhibitor therapy, which often requires enlisting the nursing staff to control systolic blood pressure in the 85 to 95 mm Hg range. This effort often requires some inservice training for a nursing staff not accustomed to dealing with advanced heart failure. The nursing staff should be instructed to reduce diuretic exposure rather than withhold ACE inhibitors for moderate hypotension. Hospitalization should also include an attempt to minimize diuretic therapy for most patients. Extensive clinical data document that intensive diuretic therapy over time tends to increase renin–angiotensin activity; this complicates ACE inhibitor therapy. A brief period of inotropic support and reduction of diuretics often enables the clinician to significantly enhance ACE inhibitor doses. The patient should clearly understand dietary salt and water limitations and the importance of accurately checking his or her early morning weight daily for adjusting diuretic doses.

The physician should document risk–benefit issues, particularly in regard to anticoagulants and amiodarone, and should discuss the risk of sudden death with the patient and family. Finally, the discharging physician should consider referring the patient for participation in clinical trials, since most trials now require a good program of baseline therapy and offer patients with advanced heart failure some hope and support with an otherwise extraordinarily depressing disease.

Consultations with ancillary providers offer many advantages. Often the physician cannot take the time to offer the expertise that ancillary providers do. Social service and clinical psychology consultations may offer substantial help with the devastating effect of heart failure on both individual and family. A reassessment of disability status, help with expensive drugs, and counseling about appropriate levels of situational anxiety and depression can all be covered by ancillary providers. Financial counseling from the health care provider may reduce worries about the expense of illness as well. Consultation with a member of the clergy may help the patient clarify his or her thinking about advance directives. In general, patients and family should be aware of the potential for sudden and unexpected death in advanced heart failure and should be advised to have a valid advance directive on file with their health care providers.

Heart failure patients and their families, particularly the primary meal provider, should have an in-depth meeting with a dietitian who understands the appropriate salt and water limitations. Most patients do not initially grasp the concept of overall daily fluid intake. Many individuals who are told to limit their water intake continue to consume large quantities of ice, juices, or carbonated beverages. An experienced dietitian can help convert refractory heart failure to ambulatory class II heart failure through education.

When available, consultation with a clinical pharmacist may be helpful to review the risks and benefits of various drugs and assess the possibility of drug interactions. For example, pharmacists may point out sodium retention and azotemia from nonsteroidal anti-inflammatory drugs when they review both prescription and over-the-counter drug intake with patients at discharge.

Cardiac rehabilitation programs focused on heart failure can help reduce the symptoms of heart failure and improve exercise tolerance. Almost all heart failure patients can undergo some degree of successful rehabilitation. Finally, home health services plays an important role for almost all patients. Much of the information given at hospital discharge is lost unless reinforced. A qualified home health nurse who sees the patient and family in follow-up in the home environment can identify and review these critical issues. Home health nurses can also assess the patient's response to outpatient management and recommend measures to forestall readmission.

THE OFFICE FOLLOW-UP CHECKLIST

Office follow up visits for heart failure patients include more than adjustment of diuretic therapy. One useful mnemonic for a complete office follow up is REPAIR (Fig. 15.3). The goals of this visit include optimal management of the patient's home environment, medica-

R: Review the patient's instructions; review diet, activity, drugs with particular attention to salt and water management.

E: Evaluate any changes in cardiac status; Has *anything* changed since last visit?

P: Pharmacologic review: Are the doses of ACE inhibitors adequate? Could we cut back on the diuretic dose? Are other drugs, prescription or over the counter, a problem?

A: Arrhythmia check: Palpitations, rapid or slow heart rates, lightheaded or "dizzy" spells. If atrial fibrillation is present, should we attempt cardioversion or offer other intervention?

I: Investigate for other problems that could mimic cardiac symptoms; particularly anemia or pulmonary disease. Check renal function, electrolytes, and thyroid function.

R: Rehabilitate! Continuing efforts to rehabilitate are critical for patients who find activity difficult. Encourage family support for the process.

Figure 15.3:   A mnemonic for the heart failure patient's follow-up office visit.

tions, and rehabilitation efforts, as well as a continued effort on the part of the medical care provider to look at the whole patient.

The review of patient instructions should include a detailed inquiry into diet, activity, and drugs. Encourage the patient to bring his or her medications and whatever written memory aids are used at home to the office. Going over this material provides a double benefit. First, the medical care provider has the opportunity to identify and correct any errors or discrepancies. Second, patients and their families realize that these issues are important and that the medical care provider is seriously interested in the program at home.

Next, an interim history and physical offers the opportunity to evaluate any changes in cardiac status. Has anything changed since the last visit, either better or worse, and if so why? The pharmacological review is an internal dialogue for the physician. The physician must ask if the drug doses are adequate; if he or she continue to up titrate the ACE inhibitor; if β-adrenergic blockade should be initiated or continued, and if any of the drug doses should be reduced.

The arrhythmia check confirms the intimate relationship between mechanical cardiac dysfunction, neurohumoral activation, and cardiac arrhythmia. The heart failure state is highly arrhythmogenic, and arrhythmia markedly exacerbates heart failure. Unfortunately, particularly with atrial fibrillation, what one sees in the office is not what one gets at home. Any unexplained changes in functional capacity or state of compensation should prompt ambulatory monitoring. Patients with atrial fibrillation are particularly at risk for intermittent tachycardia or bradycardia, and most should be considered as candidates for electrophysiologic consultation.

Next, particularly if symptomatic deterioration is not clearly explained by worsening cardiac status, other medical problems that either mimic or affect cardiac disease should be investigated. Coexistent primary cardiac and pulmonary disease, which frequently results from long-standing tobacco abuse, is probably the most difficult problem in this area. Patients who have heart failure and symptomatic chronic lung disease are particularly challenging when they complain increasing shortness of breath. An outpatient right heart catheterization, generally a 20- to 30-min simple percutaneous procedure, frequently clarifies the problem.

Finally, relentlessly continued rehabilitation efforts must not be neglected. Patients often require two or three attempts at rehabilitation before they accept the idea that physical activity is actually possible. The clinician or the office nurse, should carefully ask whether other individuals, particularly family members have derailed the rehabilitation effort with well-meaning but negative comments.

The office interaction offers a rich opportunity to interact with the patient and family in a setting in which the patient's attention is not diverted by the multiple distractions of an inpatient admission. The items listed in the REPAIR checklist easily fit into the format of a 15- to 20-min office visit. Office visits that follow the checklist become smoother, more effective, and more comprehensive than do more free-wheeling interactions.

SUMMARY

In summary, the checklist approach to these well-defined situations in heart failure care offers a method for carefully assessing and carefully managing the patient. The approach does not offer cookbook solutions but provides a comprehensive overview of management that enables the physician to feel comfortable that he or she has addressed all the relevant issues for high-quality continuing care.

SUGGESTED READING

ACC/AHA Task Force. Guidelines for the evaluation and management of heart failure. J Am Coll Cardiol 1995;26:1376–1398.

Young JB, Farmer JA. The diagnostic evaluation of patients with heart failure. In: Hosenpud JD, Greeberg BH, eds., Congestive heart failure: pathophysiology, diagnosis, and comprehensive approach to management. New York: Springer-Verlag, 1994:597–621.

Section 3

The Role of Surgery in Heart Failure Therapy

Issues for Primary Caregivers and Gatekeepers

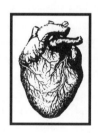

Chapter 16

Surgical Therapies for Heart Failure

Nicholas G. Smedira, Patrick M. McCarthy, and James B. Young

Many surgical procedures can ameliorate specific cardiac difficulties that lead to heart failure. Coronary artery bypass surgery and valvular repair or replacement focus on pathologic states that precipitate ventricular dysfunction if left untreated. Other approaches, e.g., ventricular volume reduction surgery and cardiomyoplasty, address the results of contractile dysfunction and heart failure, such as cardiac dilatation. As many as 40,000 to 70,000 Americans are potential candidates for cardiac transplantation, but only 2 to 5% of this population undergoes the procedure annually (1). Unless major strides expand the donor heart pool, no significant increase in the number of cardiac transplant procedures will occur. The marked disparity between donor supply and demand and the limitation of suitable alternatives to transplantation have driven a concerted effort to investigate newer surgical treatments of heart failure and redefine indications for many standard operations. More radical procedures are considered only when the patient has not responded to optimal medical therapy and when conventional surgical approaches, such as the coronary artery bypass graft (CABG), are not appropriate. Table 16.1 lists the broad spectrum of surgical alternatives for patients with heart failure.

SURGICAL REVASCULARIZATION

Coronary revascularization is the most important operative intervention to consider in patients with heart failure. Indeed, the most commonly performed operation to treat heart failure is CABG. Patients with asymptomatic left ventricular dysfunction (LVD), com-

Table 16.1.   Surgical Procedures to Consider When Treating Patients with Heart Failure

High-risk standard operative procedures
- Coronary artery bypass grafting
- Valve repair or replacement
- Left ventricular aneurysmectomy or endoaneurysmorrophy

Procedures for patients with acute heart failure
- Postinfarction revascularization for acutely stunned, hibernating, or ischemic myocardium
- Ventricular septal defect closure
- Mitral valve replacement or repair for acute mitral regurgitation (flail mitral leaflet or ruptured papillary muscle)
- Ventricular pseudoaneurysm repair
- Urgent valve repair or replacement for acute valvular insufficiency during endocarditis

Emerging operative options
- Dynamic cardiomyoplasty (cardiac wrap, extracardiac pump wrap, or aortic conduit wrap)
- Partial left ventriculectomy (ventricular reduction or remodeling surgery)
- Long-term ventricular assist devices (as bridge or alternative to transplantation)
- Total artificial heart implantation (as bridge to transplantation)

---

pensated congestive heart failure (CHF), overt CHF, chronic end-stage heart failure, and acute cardiogenic shock may benefit. Coronary heart disease, either isolated or coupled with hypertension, is the most common cause of ventricular dysfunction. Relief of active ischemia is associated with clinical improvement and improvement in heart failure morbidity and mortality.

Most clinical trials today that enroll an unselected heart failure population have a predominance of patients with coronary artery disease (CAD). In the Studies of Left Ventricular Dysfunction (SOLVD) Trials, 38% of patients had angina pectoris and 66% had a previous myocardial infarction (MI) (2). The risk of developing overt symptomatic CHF increases twofold to threefold in patients with angina pectoris and fourfold to sixfold in patients with prior MI. In the Framingham Study, coronary heart disease alone was the second most common identifiable problem causing heart failure, after hypertension (3). Hypertension is a significant risk factor for the development of CAD and is intimately linked to obstructive coronary lesions, which set the stage for acute myocardial infarction or chronic ischemic syndromes (4).

A large number of patients with both asymptomatic left ventricular systolic dysfunction and clinical CHF have potentially reversible areas of myocardial ischemia. The U.S. Department of Health and Human Services, Agency for Health Care Policy and Research (AHCPR) focused particular attention on this issue (5). The AHCPR guidelines point out three heart failure patient sets who should be evaluated for CAD: *(a)* patients with angina pectoris, *(b)* patients with a history of prior MI but no current angina, and *(c)* patients who had neither angina nor a past history of MI but who were at risk for ischemic heart disease. Note that patients who have suffered prior MI may have large areas of viable muscle in the region of the infarction or ischemic regions supplied by other coronary arteries that have disease amenable to revascularization procedures. Almost half of the patients suffering an acute MI have significant ischemia in distributions of other nonindex infarct coronary arteries (6). Some of these ischemic zones could be characterized as silent. Correction of this silent myocardial ischemia, in addition to relieving more symptomatic ischemia, may prevent deterioration of ventricular function.

Benefits of Coronary Artery Bypass Grafting

In patients with left ventricular systolic dysfunction and heart failure associated with CAD with ischemia, the goal of revascularization is to prevent further ischemic injury to the remaining functional myocardium and to restore function to hibernating regions of the left ventricle. *Hibernating myocardium* describes nonfunctional myocardial wall segments that are hypoperfused but still viable, distinct from scar or ischemia. Survival in patients with LVD is correlated to the degree of active ischemia or hibernation present. Patients without ischemia or hibernation who demonstrate only postinfarct scar are unlikely to benefit from revascularization procedures.

Unfortunately, no randomized clinical trials have specifically evaluated the outcome of CABG surgery in patients with heart failure. The three large randomized clinical trials of CABG surgery versus medical management specifically excluded patients with clinically significant congestive heart failure and left ventricular dysfunction, defined as an ejection fraction (EF) less than 35% (7–9). However, cohort studies that evaluated the effect of CABG surgery on survival in patients with heart failure and severe angina pectoris have shown positive results (9–18). Coronary artery bypass graft surgery provides its greatest survival advantage in patients with heart failure who also have angina pectoris. Table 16.2 summarizes the clinical trials reported by AHCPR to support its recommendation for CABG surgery.

It is important to recognize both classic angina pectoris and angina equivalents in heart failure, since ischemia can manifest as dyspnea on exertion or even acute pulmonary edema. Many diabetics exhibit silent myocardial ischemia (17,18), but the measure of ischemia required when symptoms are not present is not well characterized (19,20).

Risks of CABG Surgery

Although patients with heart failure benefit from revascularization, ejection fraction remains an important predictor of operative mortality (21,22). Recent reports suggest that EF has fallen from first to fourth most important adverse outcome predictor (following repeat CABG surgery, emergent CABG surgery, and age) (21). Compared to patients who have an EF greater than 40%, those whose EF is less than 20% had a threefold to fourfold higher chance of dying in the perioperative period (22). Early postoperative mortality of about 12% has been reported in patients with an EF less than 20% (21,22), although this experience is now more than a decade old. Elefteriades et al. (23) more recently summarized a single-surgeon, single-center experience in patients with left ventricular EF less than 30% and suggested hospital mortality should now be closer to 5%. In 135 consecutive patients with ejection fractions from 10 to 30% (mean = 24%), angina class improved, left ventricular EF generally rose, and 3-year survival was 81%.

Important additional determinants of mortality after CABG surgery include: age, which increases risk approximately 0.5% per year above the age of 60, gender (women have higher risk), diabetes, significant renal dysfunction, significant obstructive pulmonary disease, and significant cerebral vascular disease. And in addition, prior cardiothoracic surgery, need for emergent CABG surgery (usually

Table 16.2.   Cohort Studies of CABG Versus Medical Management for Patients with Heart Failure or Reduced EF and CAD

Study Years	Inclusion Criteria	Group	Number	Average Age, years	Percentage with Clinical Heart Failure	Percentage with Limiting Angina	Mean Ejection Fraction, %	Operative Mortality, %	Follow-up, years	Totality Mortality	Absolute Mortality Difference,%[a]	Reference
1968–1972	EF < 25%	Medical	42	55	50	76	19	NA	1.0	31	−19	16
		Surgical	24	51				33		50		
1968–1971	Depressed left ventricular function	Medical	155	55	60	100	29	NA	6.0	68	25	12
		Surgical	246	54	56	100	24	14		43		
1969–1975	EF < 30%	Medical	70	56	66	74	20	NA	2.0	53	30	11
		Surgical	46	56	43	98	21	4		23		
1966–1972	EF < 25%	Medical	21	52	NR	100	NR	NA	2.0	67	7	14
		Surgical	10				NR	NR		60		
1970–1977	EF < 35%	Medical	115	54	26	37	25	NA	5.0	66	29	13
		Surgical	77	54	21	65	27	1.3		37		
1975–1979	EF ≤ 35%	Medical	420	54	19	51	26	NA	3.0	33	10	9
		Surgical	231	56	11	72	27	7		23		
1969–1974	Clinical heart failure	Medical	44	53	100	(82)	NR	NA	6.0	Hazard ratio: 0.85	NA	15
		Surgical	83	54	100	(96)	NR	NR				
1976–1983	EF ≤ 40%	Medical	409	54	NR	NR	29	NA	3.0	32	18	10
		Surgical	301	55	NR	NR	33	NR		14		

Modified from Konstam M, Dracup K, Baker D, et al. Heart failure: evaluation and care of patients with left-ventricular systolic dysfunction [Clinical practice guideline No. 11; AHCPR Publication 94-0612]. Rockville, MD: Agency for Health Care Policy and Research, June 1994.
NA, not applicable; *NR*, not reported.
[a] Medical − surgery mortality.

in the setting of a failed percutaneous transluminal coronary angioplasty attempt or acute MI), and concomitant valvular heart surgery increase operative mortality (21,22).

Percutaneous Transluminal Coronary Angioplasty Interventions

Percutaneous transluminal coronary angioplasty (PTCA) intervention procedures are often considered to be alternatives to CABG surgery. These less-invasive approaches to revascularization have improved remarkably over the past decade, and there has been significant diminution in procedure risks and restenosis rates. No randomized clinical trials have addressed survival after PTCA compared to CABG surgery or standard medical management in heart failure cohorts. Several case series suggest that PTCA can effectively resolve angina and improve ventricular function or ischemia-induced wall motion abnormalities (24–27). Many issues must be considered when deciding to perform CABG surgery or PTCA, including patient preferences and technical challenges created by an individual's coronary anatomy.

AHCPR Recommendations

Final AHCPR recommendations suggest that heart failure patients without contraindications to surgery who have exercise-limiting angina, angina pectoris occurring frequently at rest, or recurrent episodes of acute pulmonary edema in a setting of diminished ejection fraction, should undergo coronary artery angiography as the initial diagnostic test. Selected patients may need subsequent physiologic testing to quantitate ischemic myocardium or determine myocardial viability. On the other hand, heart failure patients without significant angina pectoris after MI should undergo physiologic testing followed by coronary angiography if ischemic regions are identified. In patients without prior MI or significant chest pain, the decision to employ physiologic tests for ischemia versus coronary angiography should be based on each individual's risk for coronary heart disease and the likelihood of alternative causes for the heart failure (alcoholic cardiomyopathy, hypertensive heart disease, or valvular heart disease). Physiologic testing and coronary angiography together allow a reasonable estimate of the risks and benefits of revascularization.

VALVULAR HEART DISEASE

Valvular heart disease still represents a challenging problem. When operative timing is appropriate, surgery may prevent the development of CHF (28). The remarkable improvement in the outcome of surgery for valvular heart disease over the past two decades is likely owing to better timing of surgical intervention along with improvement in prosthetic valves, better myocardial preservation techniques, and minimally invasive surgical techniques. Significant valvular lesions alter the hemodynamics for the left or right ventricle (or both), which leads to mechanical dysfunction, muscle hypertrophy, chamber dilation (remodeling), and subsequent heart failure.

Aortic Stenosis

Aortic stenosis remains asymptomatic for extraordinarily long periods of time, but when angina, syncope, or heart failure appears, deterioration is rapid and survival is markedly compromised. Indeed, once symptoms develop, 50% of patients who do not undergo surgery die within 2 to 5 years. There is no medical therapy for this malady. Percutaneous valvuloplasty might be a reasonable alternative in patients too frail to undergo a major open-heart surgical procedure; however, balloon aortic valvuloplasty is only a palliative approach. The rate of death, cerebral vascular accidents, aortic rupture, or substantive new aortic regurgitation is in excess of 10% in many series; and mortality rates are reported to be 60% at 18 months, similar to mortality rates in untreated populations. Aortic balloon valvuloplasty as a bridging procedure in critically ill patients, with severe hepatic and renal impairment precipitated by advanced heart failure may stabilize some individuals who can subsequently undergo surgical intervention at much less risk.

Patients with aortic stenosis and significant pressure gradients generally have marked symptomatic improvement after aortic valve replacement. For patients with low transaortic valve pressure gradients in a setting of a low ejection fraction, persistent symptoms after surgery and higher mortality rates complicate the decision to operate. Typically, an aortic valve gradient of more than 50 mm Hg or valve area of less than 0.8 cm/m^2 indicates critical aortic stenosis. Pressure gradients may not adequately reflect the severity of the valve lesion, however, when severe heart failure is present. Echocardiography may allow more precise assessment of the significance of the lesion. In individuals with compromised systolic left ventricular function, surgical outcomes are better if both the cardiac output and the aortic valve pressure gradient increase significantly after either inotropic or nitroprusside infusion.

When associated coronary atherosclerosis with obstructive lesions leads to MI or chronic ischemic syndromes, the combination of aortic valve replacement and CABG procedures has proved highly beneficial in selected patients, although mortality rates are higher. Patients with large areas of left ventricular scar are not likely to improve significantly after surgery, and every attempt should be made to quantify the severity of the aortic valve lesion, coronary obstruction, and degree of left ventricular scar, ischemia, and myocardial hibernation.

Mitral Stenosis

Mitral stenosis patients generally have normal systolic left ventricular function; their symptoms are typical of heart failure as a result of diastolic dysfunction with dyspnea on exertion, orthopnea, and paroxysmal nocturnal dyspnea. Occasionally, hemoptysis, hoarseness, and symptoms of right-sided heart failure occur secondary to either concomitant tricuspid valve disease or severe pulmonary hypertension. Uncontrolled atrial fibrillation often contributes to heart failure in these patients as well.

The medical therapy of mitral stenosis focuses on preventing infective endocarditis, reducing left atrial pressure, controlling atrial fibrillation, and preventing embolic episodes. For moderate symptoms, particularly when pulmonary hypertension is present, surgical or balloon valvuloplasty is indicated. In contradistinction to balloon valvuloplasty for aortic stenosis, this procedure sometimes provides excellent long-term mechanical relief and substantive symptomatic improvement in patients with mitral stenosis. Heavily calcified valves, severe submitral valve anatomic distortion, and concomitant significant mitral regurgitation favor surgery. The alternative approaches include open commissurotomy, valve reconstruction, and mitral valve replacement.

Mitral Regurgitation

Nonischemic mitral regurgitation is most often caused by infective endocarditis, myxomatous degeneration of the mitral valve, spontaneous rupture of chordae tendineae, collagen vascular disease, and rheumatic fever. Chronic mitral regurgitation is also associated with cardiac remodeling characterized by ventricular hypertrophy, ventricular dilation, and atrial enlargement. Unless mitral regurgitation is acute and massive, the lesion usually progresses in an insidious fashion, causing significant ventricular dysfunction before symptoms of heart failure are noted.

Patients presenting with asymptomatic left ventricular systolic dysfunction owing to mitral valvular insufficiency should have the lesion corrected. Once the EF has fallen below 60% in a setting of significant mitral regurgitation, long-term prognosis is poor. Similarly, when the end-systolic dimension exceeds 4.5 cm, the prognosis is not good. Other adverse prognostic indicators include right ventricular dysfunction associated with pulmonary hypertension. Patients with a right ventricular EF less than 30% are believed to be at significant risk of an adverse event. As with aortic stenosis, concomitant CAD complicates the picture, and the relative contributions of valvular insufficiency and coronary heart disease, particularly when heart failure is present, need to be clarified.

Mitral valve repair is the preferred procedure in patients with mitral regurgitation. Mitral valve repair has a lower operative mortality and better long-term result than does mitral valve replacement. More controversial is the isolated repair of the mitral valve in patients with dilated cardiomyopathy and concomitant mitral regurgitation secondary to distortion of the valve anatomy. Some reports suggest that this can be a reasonable option in patients with severely reduced left ventricular ejection fraction (29).

Aortic Regurgitation

Aortic regurgitation is generally caused by infective endocarditis, rheumatic fever, or a degenerating bicuspid aortic valve. Disease of the aortic root owing to Marfan syndrome, aortic dissection, collagen vascular disease, and rarely syphilis can also cause regurgitation. As with mitral regurgitation, left ventricular remodeling develops insidiously over the course of many years. Left ventricular enlargement produces a large forward stroke volume that is entirely ejected through the aortic valve, in contrast to mitral regurgitation, in which the regurgitant volume enters the left atrium. Significant aortic regurgitation results in systolic hypertension with a concomitant left ventricular afterload increase. Afterload in severe aortic regurgitation can be as high as in critical aortic stenosis. Symptoms of left-sided heart failure include dyspnea, orthopnea, and fatigue. Angina may be present without concomitant obstructive coronary disease but less frequently than in patients with aortic stenosis. Aortic insufficiency should be addressed surgically when symptoms develop. There is also justification for correcting significant but asymptomatic aortic regurgitation to prevent ventricular remodeling. Because relief of aortic insufficiency dramatically decreases afterload, ventricular size often diminishes significantly with a rise in ejection fraction. Generally, when the left ventricular systolic EF falls below 50 or 55% and the left ventricular internal end-systolic dimension increases to 5 or 5.5 cm, surgery should be performed. If the EF falls below 20 to 30%, postoperative complications rise. There is some suggestion that an increased ejection fraction and decreased left ventricular volume in response to inotropic agents or exercise will predict improved outcome after aortic valve repair or replacement, despite left ventricular systolic dysfunction.

Acute aortic insufficiency is a surgical emergency. The sudden regurgitant volume presented to the left ventricle cannot be compensated, and left ventricular filling pressure rises dramatically, causing acute pulmonary edema. Reduced forward flow quickly causes coronary artery insufficiency, which further contributes to impaired ventricular function. Cardiogenic shock develops rapidly and the mortality is high. Common causes of acute aortic insufficiency include infective endocarditis, aortic dissection, and sudden perivalvular leak in a patient who has had prior aortic valve replacement.

Acute Heart Failure after MI

Acute MI may cause heart failure most appropriately managed by urgent surgical intervention (30). Surgically treatable causes of postinfarction shock include papillary muscle rupture with acute mitral regurgitation, ventricular septal defect, free wall rupture with pericardial effusion and cardiac tamponade, and left ventricular pseudoaneurysm formation. Cardiogenic shock precipitated without other mechanical impairment may respond to acute revascularization, but confirmation of the presence of significant ongoing ischemia or hibernating or stunned myocardium is mandatory.

Left ventricular free wall rupture and postinfarction ventricular septal defects occur in approximately 5% of acute myocardial infarctions in the first week. Left ventricular free wall rupture, unless contained by the pericardium, is invariably fatal. Urgent surgical repair is mandatory for patient survival. A pseudoaneurysm should also be considered an indication for emergent surgical intervention, regardless of size. Ventricular septal defect occurring post-MI is also associated with a high mortality, if the lesion is not repaired. Sudden hemodynamic compromise generally develops with a new systolic murmur. Delay in surgery is associated with high mortality; urgent surgical intervention is the preferred approach. Acute mitral regurgitation after MI may also be seen in as many as 5% of patients, more commonly with circumflex or dominant right coronary artery lesions and rupture of the posteromedial papillary muscle in 80% of cases. Early surgical intervention is warranted.

The decision to insert mechanical left ventricular assist devices to support primary pump failure caused by the infarcted, ischemic, or hibernating myocardial tissue generally commits the patient to cardiac transplantation. Smaller, impeller-driven nonpulsatile ventricular assist devices that are less complicated to insert are being developed. Because these machines are easier to remove, or can simply be shut down, we may see more frequent use of peri-infarct ventricular assist technology as a bridge to recovery instead of a bridge to transplant. Still, a thorough search for reparable lesions is important before making a decision for this aggressive form of postinfarction hemodynamic resuscitation.

DYNAMIC CARDIOMYOPLASTY

Dynamic cardiomyoplasty was introduced into clinical practice more than a decade ago as a potential alternative to cardiac transplantation. It entails mobilization of the latissimus dorsi muscle (most commonly the left) and placing it into the mediastinum, while maintaining integrity of the proximal neurovascular pedicle. The muscle is wrapped around the heart, and pacing-sensing electrodes are placed into the skeletal muscle and myocardium. The skeletal muscle is then trained with the myostimulating pacemaker for 6 to 8 weeks after surgery. Anecdotal reports suggest improvement in symptoms with modest increases in left ventricular EF. No significant change in peak oxygen consumption has been demonstrated, and the lack of substantive change in hemodynamic variables or improvement in long-term survival compared to medical therapy has polarized opinion regarding the procedure.

Recently, Bocchi et al. (31) compared cardiac transplantation, cardiomyoplasty, and medical therapy in a nonrandomized study. At 12-month follow-up, event-free survival was 79% with cardiomyoplasty and 78% with transplantation; and at 24 months, survival was 62% with cardiomyoplasty and 69% with transplantation. The survival rate with transplantation in this study was lower than that noted in most cardiac transplant centers.

Furnary et al. (32) reported a multicenter, nonrandomized trial of dynamic cardiomyoplasty in New York Heart Association (NYHA) class III patients with various causes of heart disease. Postoperative mortality was 12%, and 12-month survival 68%. Improvements were noted in NYHA class, daily living activity scores, and left ventricular EF; but no objective improvement was found in peak oxygen consumption, pulmonary capillary wedge pressure, or heart rates.

Magovern et al. (33) characterized patients who were at high risk of adverse outcome after cardiomyoplasty. Patients with substantive biventricular CHF, pulmonary hypertension, and elevated pulmonary vascular resistance had a 40% surgical mortality. The best outcomes were in patients with EF greater than 20%, preserved right ventricular function, normal sinus rhythm, normal pulmonary vascular resistance, no significant impairment in pulmonary function, and no significant ventricular arrhythmias. These authors also noted that clinical symptoms improved in patients undergoing cardiomyoplasty, but by 21 months after surgery, one-third of the patients had died.

Morerira et al. (34) examined the results of 112 patients who underwent surgery in Latin America between 1987 and 1994. Actuarial survival rates were 78.4% at 1 year, 59.7% at 2 years, and 41.7% at 5 years. Sudden cardiac death caused 38% of the late deaths; the remaining late deaths were caused by heart failure progression.

Dynamic cardiomyoplasty often improves symptoms of heart failure, but without positive physiologic changes. Mechanisms proposed to explain the benefit of the procedure include *(a)* a girdling effect, which provides passive diastolic restraint to the myocardium, preventing further ventricular dilation and remodeling; and *(b)* physiologic hypertrophy provided by the additive muscle wrap, which reduces left ventricular free wall stress, subsequently diminishing myocardial oxygen demand. Whether dynamic cardiomyoplasty prolongs survival compared to medically treated groups is uncertain, and a randomized prospective study has been initiated. Patients appear to do best when they have mild to moderate heart failure; therefore, this procedure may not be an alternative to cardiac transplantation but a procedure to attenuate heart failure that should be considered before heart transplant.

PARTIAL LEFT VENTRICULECTOMY

Partial left ventricular resection (volume reduction surgery), generally with mitral valve repair, is a novel surgical approach to patients with medically refractory heart failure and substantive ventricular dilation (35–38). This procedure consists of removal of a section of the left ventricular myocardium (usually the interpapillary muscle region) and repair of concomitant regurgitant mitral valve lesions. The goal of the operation is to reduce ventricular chamber diameter and eliminate mitral regurgitation. The rationale is based on the Laplace's law, which states that the average circumferential wall stress of the heart is directly proportional to the intraventricular pressure and radius of the ventricular at the endocardial surface and indirectly related to the wall thickness.

The operation reduces the diameter of the left ventricle, increasing wall thickness and reducing intraventricular pressure to reduce wall stress. Patients with dilated cardiomyopathy and normal coronary anatomy fair best. Initial experience suggests that at least 25% of patients subjected to the operation improve significantly, and another 50% of patients see some, albeit less-impressive, benefit. There is an overall 5 to 10% mortality, and 20 to 25% of the patients require alterative backup support strategies, such as assist devices or transplantation. By selecting patients who would be candidates for cardiac transplantation, the surgeon can rationalize the operation. Refinement of surgical technique, criteria predictive of positive outcomes, and documentation of beneficial long-term results will dictate appropriate practice with time.

PERMANENT LEFT VENTRICULAR ASSIST DEVICE IMPLANTATION

Long-term left ventricular assist device implantation is not yet an accepted alternative to cardiac transplantation; however, some initial experience has been reported (39–42). Significant improvement in exercise and hemodynamic status can be achieved with these remarkable systems. A randomized study began in 1996 to compare advanced heart failure medical therapy to the HeartMate™ (ThermoCardiosystems, Inc., Woburn, MA) left ventricular assist device. Patients entering this protocol do not meet conventional criteria for cardiac transplantation owing to comorbidities. This study will provide definitive data concerning long-term performance of these pumps.

SUMMARY

Medical and surgical teamwork offers an interdependent strategy for heart failure management. Selected operative interventions may dramatically improve long-term prognosis and decrease heart failure symptoms, morbidity, and mortality. The search for procedures that might serve as alternatives to cardiac transplantation continues. Although no alternative to cardiac transplantation exists today, standard operative procedures—albeit associated with higher risks— may offer satisfactory approaches for many heart transplantation patients. We do not have adequate information regarding survival of patients with more profound left ventricular systolic dysfunction who undergo dynamic cardiomyoplasty or partial left ventricular resection. There is the suggestion, however, that symptoms and morbidity decrease after these operations. Partial left ventricular resection and chronic ventricular assist devices are evolving technologies about to enter the clinical trials arena.

REFERENCES

1. Young JB, Frost A, Short HD. A clinical perspective of heart and lung transplantation. Immunol Clin North Am 1996;16:265–291.
2. Effect of enalapril on survival in patients with reduced left ventricular ejection fractions and congestive heart failure. The SOLVD investigators. N Engl J Med 1991;325:293–302.
3. Ho KK, Pinsky JL, Kannel WB, Levy D. The epidemiology of heart failure: the Framingham Study. J Am Coll Cardiol 1993;22:6A–13A.

4. Kannel WB, Levy D, Cupples LA. Left ventricular hypertrophy and risk of cardiac failure: insights from the Framingham Study. J Cardiovasc Pharmacol 1987;10:S135–S140.
5. Konstam M, Dracup K, Baker D, et al. Heart failure: evaluation and care of patients with left-ventricular systolic dysfunction [Clinical practice guideline No. 11; AHCPR Publication 94-0612]. Rockville, MD: Agency for Health Care Policy and Research, June 1994.
6. Kotler TS, Diamond GA. Exercise thallium-201 scintigraphy in the diagnosis and prognosis of coronary artery disease. Ann Intern Med 1990;113:684–702.
7. Murphy ML, Hultgren HN, Detre K, et al. Treatment of chronic stable angina: a preliminary report of the randomized Veterans Administration Cooperative Study. N Engl J Med 1977;297:621–627.
8. Varnauskas E. Twelve-year follow-up of survival in the randomized European Coronary Surgery Study. N Engl J Med 1988;319:332–337.
9. Alderman EL, Fisher LD, Litwin P, et al. Results of coronary artery surgery in patients with poor left ventricular function (CASS). Circulation 1983;68:785–795.
10. Bounous EP, Mark DB, Pollock BG, et al. Surgical survival benefits for coronary disease patients with left-ventricular dysfunction. Circulation 1988;78:I151–I157.
11. Faulkner SL, Stoney WS, Alford WC, et al. Ischemic cardiomyopathy: medical versus surgical treatment. J Thorac Cardiovasc Surg 1977;74:77–82.
12. Manley JC, King JF, Zeft HJ, et al. The "bad" left ventricle: results of coronary surgery and effect on late survival. J Thorac Cardiovasc Surg 1976;72:841–848.
13. Pigott JD, Kouchoukos NT, Oberman A, et al. Late results of medical and surgical therapy for patients with coronary artery disease and depressed ejection fraction [Abstract]. Circulation 1982;66(Suppl 2):II220.
14. Vliestra RE, Assad-Morell JL, Frye RL, et al. Survival predictors in coronary artery disease. Medical and surgical comparisons. Mayo Clin Proc 1977;52:85–90.
15. Hammermeister KE, DeRouen TA, Doge HT. Comparison of survival of medically and surgically treated coronary disease patients in Seattle Heart Watch: a nonrandomized study. Circulation 1982;65(Part 2):53–59.
16. Yatteau RP, Peter RH, Behar VS, et al. Ischemic cardiomyopathy: the myopathy of coronary artery disease. Natural history and results of medical versus surgical treatment. Am J Cardiol 1974;34:520–525.
17. Pratt CM, McMahon EP, Goldstein S, et al. Comparison of subgroups assigned to medical regimens used to suppress cardiac ischemia (the Asymptomatic Cardiac Ischemia Pilot ACIP Study). Am J Cardiol 1996;77:1302–1309.
18. Conti CR, Geller NL, Knatterud GL, et al. Anginal status and prediction of cardiac events in patients enrolled in the Asymptomatic Cardiac Ischemia Pilot (ACIP) study. ACIP Investigators. Am J Cardiol 1997;79:889–892.
19. Brunken R, Schwaiger M, Grover-McKay M, et al. Positron emission tomography detects tissue metabolic activity in myocardial segments with persistent thallium perfusion defects. J Am Coll Cardiol 1987;10:557–567.
20. Kiat H, Berman DS, Maddahi J, et al. Late reversibility of tomographic myocardial thallium-201 defects: an accurate marker of myocardial viability. J Am Coll Cardiol 1988;12:1456–1463.
21. Christakis GT, Ivanov J, Weisel RD, et al. The changing pattern of coronary artery bypass surgery. Circulation 1989;80:I151–I161.
22. Hannan EL, Kilburn H Jr, O'Donnell JF, et al. Adult open heart surgery in New York State. An analysis of risk factors and hospital mortality rates. JAMA 1990;264:2768–2774.
23. Elefteriades JA, Morales DLS, Gradel C, et al. Results of coronary artery bypass grafting by a single surgeon in patients with left ventricular ejection fractions ≤ 30%. Am J Cardiol 1997;79:1573–1578.
24. Hartzler GO, Rutherford BD, McConahay DR, et al. "High-risk" percutaneous transluminal coronary angioplasty. Am J Cardiol 1988;61:33G–37G.

25. Reinfeld HB, Samet P, Hildner FJ. Resolution of congestive failure, mitral regurgitation, and angina after percutaneous transluminal coronary angioplasty of triple vessel disease. Cathet Cardiovasc Diagn 1985;2:273–277.
26. Taylor GJ, Rabinovich E, Mikell FL, et al. Percutaneous transluminal coronary angioplasty as palliation for patients considered poor surgical candidates. Am Heart J 1986;111:840–844.
27. Serota H, Deligonul U, Lee W, et al. Predictors of cardiac survival after percutaneous transluminal coronary angioplasty in patients with severe left ventricular dysfunction. Am J Cardiol 1991;67:367–372.
28. Carabello BA, Crawford FA. Valvular heart disease. N Engl J Med 1997; 337:22–41.
29. Starling RC. Radical alternatives to transplantation. Curr Opin Cardiol 1997;12: 166–171.
30. Milgalter E, Drinkwater DC, Laks H. Surgical therapy for acute congestive heart failure. In: Hosenpud, JD, Greenburg BH, eds., Congestive heart failure: pathophysiology, diagnosis, and comprehensive approach to management. New York: Springer-Verlag, 1994.
31. Bocchi EA, Bellotti G, Moreira LF, et al. Mid-term results of heart transplantation, cardiomyoplasty, and medical treatment of refractory heart failure caused by idiopathic dilated cardiomyopathy. J Heart Lung Transplant 1996;15:736–745.
32. Furnary AP, Jessup M, Moreira LFP. Multicenter trial of dynamic cardiomyoplasty for chronic heart failure. The American Cardiomyoplasty Group. J Am Coll Cardiol 1996;28:1175–1180.
33. Magovern GJ, Simpson KA. Clinical cardiomyoplasty: review of the ten-year United States experience. Ann Thorac Surg 1996;61:413–419.
34. Moreira LFR, Stolf NAG, Braile DM, Jantene AD. Dynamic cardiomyoplasty in South America. Ann Thorac Surg 1996;61:408–412.
35. Batista RJV, Santos JLV, Takeshita N, et al. Partial left ventriculectomy to improve left ventricular function in end-stage heart disease. J Cardiovasc Surg 1996;11:96–97.
36. McCarthy PM, Starling RC, Smedira NG, et al. Partial left ventriculectomy with valve repair as an alternative to cardiac transplantation. J Heart Lung Transplant 1997;16:41.
37. McCarthy PM. Ventricular remodeling: hype or hope? Nature Med 1996; 2:859–890.
38. Starling RC, Young JB, Scalia GM, et al. Preliminary observations with ventricular remodeling surgery for refractory congestive heart failure. J Am Coll Cardiol 1997;29:64A.
39. Farrar DJ, Hill JD, Gray LA Jr, et al. Heterotopic prosthetic ventricles as a bridge to cardiac transplantation. A multicenter study in 29 patients. N Engl J Med 1988;318:333–340.
40. Griffith BP, Kormos RL, Nastala CJ, et al. Results of extended bridge to transplantation: window into the future of permanent ventricular assist devices. Ann Thorac Surg 1996;61:396–398.
41. McCarthy PM. HeartMate implantable left ventricular assist device: bridge to transplantation and future applications. Ann Thorac Surg 1995;59:S46–S51.
42. McCarthy PM, Schmitt SK, Vargo RL, et al. Implantable LVAD infections: implications for permanent use of the device. Ann Thorac Surg 1996;61:359–365.

Chapter 17

Cardiac Transplantation

Patient Selection and Post–Heart Transplantation Management

James B. Young

Cardiac transplantation has proven a remarkable therapeutic option for advanced heart failure that is unresponsive to more conservative medical and surgical management strategies. This operation is effective in diminishing morbidity and mortality when certain comorbid processes are absent (1–6). Indeed, the United Network of Organ Sharing database (1), which contains information on more than 100,000 solid organ transplant procedures, demonstrates that about 14% overall of the organs transplanted in the last decade have been hearts. The International Heart and Lung Transplant Society Registry maintains data on more than 40,000 heart transplant procedures done since 1967.

Success (80 to 90% 1- to 2-year survival rates and 75 to 80% 5- to 10-year survival rates in some programs) rests on three extraordinarily important issues: *(a)* selecting patients with heart failure syndromes severe enough to warrant this radical surgery; *(b)* ensuring that comorbid conditions or contraindications that might compromise success after transplantation are not present; and *(c)* requiring that appropriate and compulsive patient follow-up occurs, including proper management of immunomodulating drugs and techniques.

This chapter puts cardiac transplantation into perspective and highlights the nuances of patient selection, donor identification, management, and allocation and discusses long-term posttransplant patient management.

CLINICAL PATTERNS OF CARDIAC TRANSPLANTATION

The International Heart and Lung Transplantation Society registry (5) of patients who have undergone cardiac transplant includes data from 251 clinical centers. After the introduction of more effective immunosuppressant protocols in the early 1980s, procedures increased dramatically (about 500 cardiac transplant operations were done in 1983, and approximately 3500 were performed worldwide in 1990). No significant increase has occurred since 1990, however; and we appear to have reached the limit of procedures, unless an increase in organ donation can be engineered.

In the United States, the United Network for Organ Sharing (UNOS) is the contractual agency designated by the Department of Organ Transplantation (DOT) to operate the Organ Procurement and Transplantation Network (OPTN). UNOS also operates a large transplant patient database registry, which is useful to review to gain insight into our national solid organ transplant experience. Table 17.1 places cardiac transplantation into the perspective of all solid organ transplants performed. Cardiac transplantation accounts for 10 to 15% of all solid organ transplants in the United States in the last decade. Most of the procedures performed have been orthotopic implants.

Of the 50,000 potential solid organ transplant recipients currently included on the UNOS waiting list, approximately 10% are awaiting cardiac allograft allocation. Table 17.2 summarizes many characteristics of patients undergoing cardiac transplantation. Some subtle, though important, demographic changes are apparent. Particularly notable is an increase in older recipients. For example, 51.8% of heart transplant recipients were over the age of 50 in 1988, but 57.5% were over the age of 50 in 1994. Increasing numbers of women are undergoing cardiac transplant, and more patients received hearts during hospitalization for acute heart failure decompensation. About half of the patients have heart failure owing to dilated cardiomyopathy.

CARDIAC TRANSPLANT WAITING LIST CHARACTERISTICS

As noted, at least 50,000 patients are currently listed with UNOS and awaiting organ allocation (1). In 1995, a total of 3383 patients were listed for cardiac transplantation; and as shown in Table 17.3, waiting times are increasing substantially. Table 17.4 summarizes heart donor characteristics. For example, 4845 organ donors became available in 1992 (data not shown), but only 3925 were suitable

Table 17.1. U.S. Cadaveric Solid Organ Transplants[a]

Organ	Year							
	1988	1989	1990	1991	1992	1993	1994	1995
Heart	1,675	1,703	2,092	2,091	2,171	2,297	2,345	2,360
Heart–lung	74	67	52	51	48	60	70	69
Lung	33	93	202	402	535	666	722	871
Cadaveric kidney	7,228	7,093	7,784	7,727	7,697	8,170	8,384	8,598
Liver	1,714	2,201	2,682	2,951	3,031	3,404	3,592	3,926
Pancreas	249	419	537	533	557	774	842	1,028
Totals	10,973	11,576	13,349	13,755	14,039	15,371	15,955	16,852

Modified from Annual report of the U.S. Scientific Registry of Transplant Recipients and the Organ Procurement and Transplantation Network—transplant data: 1988–1996. Bethesda, MD: US Department of Health and Human Services, 1997.

[a] Year-end data.

Table 17.2. Heart Transplant Recipient Characteristics[a]

Characteristic	Year							
	1988	1989	1990	1991	1992	1993	1994	1995
Number	1676	1705	2108	2125	2171	2297	2345	2360
Age, %								
<1	2.3	4.3	4.3	5.9	4.1	4.7	4.0	3.8
1–5	1.3	1.3	2.3	2.5	2.9	2.4	2.9	2.5
6–10	1.2	1.0	1.1	0.9	1.1	1.4	1.7	1.7
11–17	2.6	2.4	2.9	3.0	2.7	3.4	2.9	3.4
18–34	11.4	10.9	8.3	8.2	8.1	8.8	7.6	7.5
35–49	29.4	29.3	27.9	26.2	24.5	23.4	23.5	22.3
50–64	50.4	48.4	49.7	49.9	52.6	51.3	53.4	52.8
65+	1.4	2.4	3.4	3.4	3.9	4.5	4.1	6.0
Male, %	79.3	79.8	78.6	77.2	76.7	78.5	76.1	76.8
Prior heart transplant, %	3.5	2.7	2.5	2.6	3.0	2.9	3.2	2.9
Heterotopic, %	1.1	0.8	0.7	0.7	0.6	0.3	0.2	0.2
Recipient descriptions, %								
Hospitalized	14.4	6.7	8.2	6.6	8.2	5.5	2.6	2.2
ICU	26.0	24.8	30.0	23.8	22.2	22.1	5.2	1.5
ICU/life support	17.4	16.8	15.6	23.6	22.5	31.4	54.0	63.2
Not hospitalized	42.2	51.7	46.1	46.0	44.1	41.0	38.3	33.0
Diagnosis, %								
Cardiomyopathy	36.6	37.2	36.5	42.3	44.0	43.0	56.2	66.7
CAD	50.4	47.7	49.0	40.8	40.7	41.5	30.8	21.1
Congenital	4.1	6.5	7.0	8.9	7.5	8.1	7.0	6.7
VHD	5.5	4.5	4.2	3.4	2.9	2.9	2.3	2.0
Heart transplant	2.7	2.4	2.6	2.9	2.9	3.1	2.2	2.6

Modified from Annual report of the U.S. Scientific Registry of Transplant Recipients and the Organ Procurement and Transplantation Network—transplant data: 1988–1996. Bethesda, MD: US Department of Health and Human Services, 1997.

ICU, intensive care unit; CAD, coronary artery disease; VHD, valvular heart disease.

[a] Year-end data.

Table 17.3. UNOS Heart Transplant Waiting List Characteristics[a]

Characteristic	Year							
	1988	1989	1990	1991	1992	1993	1994	1995
Number	1030	1320	1788	2267	2690	2834	2933	3383
Age, %								
<1	0.6	0.5	1.2	1.1	1.2	0.9	0.8	0.2
1–5	0.4	1.4	0.6	1.2	1.0	1.2	1.6	0.5
6–10	0.3	0.2	0.3	0.4	0.4	0.6	0.5	0.9
11–17	1.3	1.0	0.9	1.2	1.4	1.5	1.9	0.8
18–34	7.7	7.1	8.4	2.5	2.3	7.8	7.8	22.6
35–49	35.3	32.6	32.0	30.2	29.2	28.5	28.2	35.4
50–64	52.2	55.0	53.1	54.7	55.3	55.0	55.1	54.6
65+	2.2	2.3	3.4	3.6	4.2	4.6	4.1	4.2
Male, %	86.1	85.5	84.7	84.1	83.5	82.0	81.4	80.7
Waiting time, %								
0–30 days	19.3	15.9	13.2	10.9	8.7	9.2	9.0	8.8
31–60 days	12.4	11.9	9.7	9.7	8.2	6.7	6.9	7.4
61–90 days	11.3	10.2	8.2	8.5	7.2	5.3	5.7	5.8
91–120 days	7.3	7.4	7.6	7.1	6.5	5.4	5.1	4.1
121–150 days	7.4	6.0	6.2	6.0	5.6	5.4	3.9	5.0
151–180 days	7.2	5.0	5.9	6.1	5.2	3.9	3.5	4.8
6–12 months	22.6	23.1	28.7	24.6	26.8	21.9	20.6	21.2
> 1 year	12.5	20.5	20.4	27.2	31.8	42.1	45.4	42.9
Deaths, %	15.0	14.1	13.1	14.5	13.1	12.2	11.4	11

Modified from Annual report of the U.S. Scientific Registry of Transplant Recipients and the Organ Procurement and Transplantation Network—transplant data: 1988–1996. Bethesda, MD: US Department of Health and Human Services, 1997.

[a] Year-end data.

Table 17.4. Heart Donor Characteristics[a]

Characteristic	1988	1989	1990	1991	1992	1993	1994	1995
Number	1785	1782	2168	2198	2247	2442	2527	2505
Age, %								
< 1	1.5	3.3	3.1	4.2	2.9	3.4	2.9	2.7
1–5	1.7	3.1	3.5	3.8	3.2	3.5		2.9
6–10	2.2	1.8	2.2	2.9	2.4	2.1		3.2
11–17	17.7	15.3	14.9	15.0	16.5	18.6	18.0	17.4
18–34	55.6	53.0	51.2	48.2	42.7	42.9	40.2	40.8
35–49	19.2	21.4	22.2	22.2	24.5	21.0	24.4	24.6
50–64	2.0	3.1	3.7	4.6	6.5	7.8	8.2	8.0
65+	0.1	0.1	0	0.1	0.3	0.7	0.7	0.3
Male, %	71.7	72.1	69.8	68.4	68.3	68.6	68.7	66.8
Cause of death, %								
MVA	39.9	34.0	33.3	30.5	25.0	26.9	29.5	33.4
GSW/SW	21.3	22.1	21.3	22.7	24.6	23.2	24.7	20.9
CVA	20.6	23.4	23.2	24.5	26.6	25.7	28.0	27.3
Head trauma	10.3	12.0	12.8	11.5	13.5	12.7	27.9	63.7
Asphyxia	1.4	2.0	2.2	3.0	2.0	2.4	1.9	8.0
Drowning	0.4	0.3	0.6	0.7	0.9	0.8	0.3	0.5
Drug overdose	1.1	0.9	0.9	0.5	0.7	0.5	0.5	0.9
CV	0.7	0.6	0.6	0.7	0.5	0.9	0.8	1.3

Modified from Annual report of the U.S. Scientific Registry of Transplant Recipients and the Organ Procurement and Transplantation Network—transplant data: 1988–1996. Bethesda, MD: US Department of Health and Human Services, 1997.

MVA, motor vehicle accident; GSW, gunshot wound; SW, stab wound; CVA, cerebrovascular accident; CV, cardiovascular.

[a] Year-end data.

multiorgan donors (81% of the overall cadaveric donor pool). Of the suitable multiorgan donors only 2247 (about 50% of the overall donor pool) became cardiac donors. This proportion has been fairly constant. Obviously, the number of candidates listed each year for cardiac transplantation far exceeds the number of available donors.

THE CARDIAC ALLOGRAFT DONOR

Brain Death

Table 17.5 details criteria necessary to make the diagnosis of brain death. No evidence of cerebral cortex function may be evident and no suggestion of brainstem activity apparent. Patients, therefore, must be in a deep coma without any evidence of cerebral receptivity. The lack of brainstem activity is confirmed by absence of light pupillary, corneal, extraocular, gag, and cough reflexes; apnea is apparent in the presence of hypercarbia. One should be able to identify the

Table 17.5.   Brain Death Criteria[a]

Absence of cerebral cortex, cerebellar, and midbrain function
- No pupillary light reflex (pupils fixed)
- No corneal reflex
- No extraocular reflex (no doll's eyes motion)
- No gag reflex
- No cough reflex
- No respirations during apnea test[b] (ventilator dependent)

Irreversibility
- Cause of death certain
- Hypothermia, hypotension, or significant metabolic perturbation addressed and reversed
- No drug intoxication or significant CNS depressant use that would mask true neurologic status
- Observations persist over time (for adults: 6 h with confirmatory tests; 12 h without; 24 h in the setting of anoxic brain injury)

Ancillary confirmatory tests (not mandatory but sometimes helpful)
- Electroencephalogram
- Radionuclide imaging of brain blood flow
- Cerebral angiography to determine CNS blood flow patterns

[a] Based on total brain death concepts.
[b] Preoxygenate with 100% F_{IO_2} for 10 min; disconnect ventilator; give oxygen at 8–12 L/min by tracheal cannula; observe for spontaneous respirations; obtain $PaCO_2$ after 10 min; if $PaCO_2 > 60$ mm Hg and no respirations have occurred, individual is apneic.

cause of central nervous system (CNS) injury, and there should be no concomitant hypothermia, hypotension, significant metabolic perturbation, drug intoxication, or significant use of CNS depressants. The clinical finding should persist over specified time intervals; and if they do, confirmatory tests to diagnose brain death are not required. Electroencephalography, radionuclide cerebral blood flow imaging, and cerebral angiography may be used, however, to help clarify confusing clinical pictures or to assist with shortening observation time periods in select circumstances. Most individual institutional policies regarding declaration of brain death and state and federal statutory regulations conform to these concepts and criteria.

Acceptable Cardiac Donors

Table 17.6 summarizes acceptable guidelines for cardiac donors and lists allografts that can be successfully used. Long-term follow-up of patients after cardiac transplantation often relates to donor-specific issues (7–11). Obviously, allograft rejection will be more intense when recipient presensitization is apparent and manifest by

Table 17.6.   Suggested Guidelines for Acceptable Cardiac Donors

- Age < 55 years (older donors are sometimes acceptable)
- Negative serologies for HIV and hepatitis (some donors who are hepatitis B or C positive may be acceptable)
- No active severe systemic infection (sepsis not apparent)
- No malignancy with a possibility of metastasis (primary brain tumors usually not problematic) or other concerning comorbid condition, such as diabetes or collagen vascular disease
- No evidence of significant cardiac disease or trauma
- Low probability of coronary atherosclerosis (donor coronary angiograms should be obtained in high-risk settings; when present, donor coronary artery disease should be minimal)
- Acceptable ventricular function without aggressive inotropic support (< 10 ng/kg/min of dopamine or combined dose of 20 μg/kg/min of dopamine and dobutamine in most situations)
- Blood type compatible with recipient
- Negative cytotoxic lymphocyte cross-match for sensitized recipients
- Donor body weight index between 75 and 125% of recipient's (size mismatch affected by recipient pulmonary hypertension; small donors might be acceptable heterotopic candidates in certain clinical situations)
- Anticipated allograft ischemia times < 4–5 h (some hearts function satisfactorily with 5–8 h of ischemic time)

a positive donor–recipient cross-match. More germane to long-term care of the heart transplant recipient are cytomegalovirus mismatch and presence of coronary artery disease in the transplanted heart. Other important considerations include donor size in relation to the recipient and presence of donor comorbidities that would increase risk of graft failure. Coexisting donor malignancy should also be excluded to eliminate the possibility of cancer transmission.

SELECTION AND REFERRAL OF POTENTIAL CARDIAC TRANSPLANT CANDIDATES

Selection of candidates is critical to both optimum donor organ use and maximization of long-term survival results (12–18). Referral of patients is based on identification of severe heart failure syndromes associated with a high mortality within 12 to 24 months (14). Symptoms should be present and difficult to control with generally available medical or surgical interventions. Significant comorbid conditions that might contribute to a negative posttransplant outcome should be sought.

As noted in Table 17.7, consensus has developed regarding indications for cardiac transplantation. Patients should be limited by cardiac disease to a maximum exercise oxygen consumption of 10 mL O_2/kg/min or less after surpassing anaerobic threshold. Maximal exertion effort and an $O_2 : CO_2$ expired gas ratio greater than 1.10 should be documented. Patients with severe ischemic heart disease who suffer disabling angina pectoris and have coronary anatomy not amenable to revascularization and individuals with recurrent, symptomatic ventricular arrhythmias refractory to all drug, ablation, and arrhythmia termination device techniques are also heart transplant candidates. Additional indications for cardiac transplantation include a maximum oxygen consumption less than or equal to 14 mL O_2/kg/min in patients with severe limitation of daily activities; recurrent unstable angina without vessels amenable to revascularization; and inability to maintain euvolia without development of renal dysfunction, despite optimal medical therapy and salt and fluid restriction. Occasionally, heart failure patients with oxygen consumption levels up to 20 mL/kg/min are reasonable candidates, but other extenuating circumstances are usually present.

Table 17.7.   Indications for Cardiac Transplantation

Patients should be considered for transplantation in the presence of:
- Significant functional limitation (NYHA classes III–IV heart failure), despite maximum medical therapy, which includes digitalis, diuretics, and vasodilators
- Refractory angina or refractory life-threatening arrhythmia cannot be addressed with more conventional therapy
- Exclusion of all surgical alternatives to transplantation, such as the following, has occurred:
    Revascularization for significant reversible ischemia
    Valve replacement for critical aortic stenosis
    Valve replacement for repair of severe mitral or aortic insufficiency

Contraindications to transplant include the following:
- Disease that might otherwise shorten life expectancy
- Patients with current substance abuse, incarceration, or psychosocial concerns
- Demonstrated noncompliance with medical suggestions
- Morbid obesity

Relative contraindications to transplantation include the following:
- Pulmonary vascular resistance > 5 Wood units after drug infusion therapy
- FEV_1 < 1L or 50% of predicted
- Serum creatinine > 3 or creatinine clearance < 25 mL/min
- Ideal body weight > 150%
- Age > 65–70 years

Evaluations should consist of the following:
- Oxygen consumption treadmill testing
- Complete hemodynamic and cardiac performance evaluation and screen for fixed pulmonary hypertension
- Evaluation of potential for revascularizable ischemic heart disease
- Exclusion of comorbidities that might exclude patient as appropriate candidate

Specific recommendations
- Definite indications
    Peak exercise oxygen use < 10 mL/kg/min
    NYHA class IV
    History of recurrent hospitalization for congestive heart failure
    Refractory ischemia with inoperable coronary artery disease and left ventricular ejection fraction < 20%
    Recurrent symptomatic ventricular arrhythmias not responding to appropriate therapies
- Probable indications
    Volume of oxygen use < 14 mg/kg/min
    NYHA class III–IV
    Recent hospitalizations for congestive heart failure
    Unstable angina not amenable to cornary artery bypass grafting or percutaneous transluminal coronary angioplasty; left ventricular ejection fraction < 30%
- Inadequate indications in and of themselves
    Volume of oxygen use > 14 mL/kg/min
    NYHA class I–II
    Left ventricular ejection fraction < 20%
    Stable, exertional angina with left ventricular ejection fraction > 20%

Table 17.7.   (Continued)

Patients listed for transplant should be re-evaluated every 6 months with the following:
- Oxygen consumption exercise testing
- Hemodynamic and clinical assessment summary
- Echocardiography
- Consultations from social worker, dietician, physical therapist, financial adviser, and psychologist/psychiatrist, and other consultant only as individually indicated
- Laboratory testing, including assessments of electrolytes, creatinine clearance, urinalysis, liver functions, and coagulation profile; serologic tests for HIV and hepatitis A, B, and C if current condition or history of hepatitis; serologic testing for cytomegalovirus, toxoplasma, histoplasmosis, rubella, varicella, Epstein-Barr virus; blood and tissue typing and human leukocyte antigen profile should be obtained only in patients selected for transplantation candidacy

---

NYHA, New York Heart Association.

When selecting candidates, clinicians must make an evaluation after optimization of medical therapies, because patients with severe decompensated heart failure can often improve dramatically with aggressive treatment. Alternative surgical procedures such as coronary artery bypass grafting, valve repair or replacement, aneurysmectomy or aneurysmorrhaphy, and possibly, partial left ventriculectomy (volume reduction or remodeling surgery) should be considered as possible alternatives to transplantation. These operations can frequently palliate the condition so that cardiac transplantation is not necessary or can be significantly delayed.

Table 17.8 summarizes the tests and procedures usually performed during a heart transplant evaluation. The evaluation focuses on four important questions: *(a)* What is the stage of the patient's heart failure syndrome? *(b)* Is it severe enough to warrant consideration for cardiac transplantation? *(c)* Are there other alterative medication protocols or procedures that can be done to ameliorate the situation? *(d)* Are there comorbid conditions that might increase the risk of a poor postoperative outcome? Though sometimes tempting, performing cardiac transplantation in individuals who have a greater likelihood of failure than success is unfair to the patient, caregivers, and society at large. The real challenge is fairly forming an opinion about each individual's risk : benefit ratio.

Table 17.8. Potential Heart Transplant Candidate Evaluation[a]

General data
- Complete medical history and physical examination
- Evaluation of psychosocial parameters known to be important during the transplant experience
- Blood chemistries, renal and hepatic functions battery, thyroid function tests
- Complete blood count, platelet count, prothrombin time, partial thromboplastin time
- Urinalysis
- 24-h urine for creatinine clearance and total protein
- Stool guaiac examination
- Nutritional status and diet history
- Mammography (for females > 40 years)
- Pap smear (for females)
- Prostate specific antigen (for males > 40 years)

Basic cardiovascular data
- Electrocardiogram
- Chest x-ray
- Peak $\dot{V}o_2$ determination
- Right heart hemodynamic evaluation
- Echocardiogram with Doppler interrogation of valves
- Left heart catheterization
- Myocardial perfusion and function scintigraphic study
- Endomyocardial biopsy

Ancillary tests (when indicated)
- Pulmonary function tests (with carbon monoxide diffusing capacity)
- Pulmonary ventilation–perfusion scan or arteriography
- Ultrasound of abdominal aorta
- Ultrasound of gallbladder
- Carotid and/or lower extremity arterial noninvasive studies
- Gastrointestinal endoscopy
- Central nervous system scanning

Immunologic data
- Blood group and Rhesus type
- Human leukocyte antigen typing
- Determination of community antibody presensitization

Infectious disease background screening data
- Hepatitis B and C serology
- Herpes virus serology
- HIV serology
- Cytomegalovirus (IgM and IgG)
- Toxoplasmosis titer
- Varicella and rubella titers
- Epstein-Barr virus (IgM and IgG) titers
- Histoplasmosis and coccidioidomycosis titers
- Venereal Disease Research Laboratory test and fluorescent treponemal antibody absorption test
- Skin testing for tuberculosis with controls of mumps, dermatophytid, histoplasmosis, coccidioidmycosis

[a] Selection of tests is tailored to the individual clinical setting.

Table 17.9 specifically lists recipient characteristics that might influence decisions regarding acceptable cardiac transplant candidacy. Patient evaluations should attempt to uncover recipient-related factors important to outcome. Some factors are intuitively obvious, such as coexistent malignant neoplasms; but others, such as a lymphoma now seemingly cured, are not clear-cut contraindications. Likewise, both very young and very old patients undergoing cardiac transplantation have lower survival rates. Some programs will not consider patients over age 60 for cardiac transplantation, whereas other programs accept candidates up to 65 or even 70 years of age. Some centers keep separate lists for older patients, allocating so-called marginal donors to these patients. Review committees often decline transplantation to patients with diabetes mellitus with end-organ damage, severe osteoporosis, morbid obesity, and severe unresponsive or fixed pulmonary hypertension.

Table 17.9.   Factors That Negatively Affect Outcome after Cardiac Transplantation

- Older and younger recipient age
- Infiltrative or inflammatory diseases (amyloid, sarcoid, lupus, erythematosis)
- Irreversible pulmonary hypertension (fixed pulmonary resistance > 5 Wood units)
- Substantive parenchymal pulmonary disease (emphysema)
- Acute pulmonary thromboembolism (particularly with parenchymal infarction and residual necrosis)
- Substantive symptomatic peripheral or cerebrovascular disease (claudication, ischemic stroke, or significant aortic aneurysm)
- Irreversible and significant renal or hepatic dysfunction
- Active peptic ulcer disease
- Symptomatic diverticulitis, cholelithiasis, cholecystitis, inflammatory bowel disease
- Diabetes mellitus with end-organ damage (significant proliferative retinopathy, proteinuria, neuropathy, or peripheral vascular disease)
- Substantive ponderosity
- Severe osteoporosis
- Active infection
- Coexistent malignant neoplasms
- Certain muscular dystrophies
- Inability to actively rehabilitate
- Psychosocial instability or substance abuse that will compromise outcome by adversely affecting treatment program compliance
- Unwillingness to undergo procedure

Critically important is addressing the specific issues that can predispose patients to heart failure decompensation (Table 17.10). Elimination of these circumstances will often improve heart failure so that further consideration of heart transplantation is unnecessary.

EXPECTED OUTCOMES AFTER CARDIAC TRANSPLANTATION

Over the past 15 years, survival after cardiac transplantation has improved dramatically; and in carefully selected patients, it clearly exceeds survival with medical therapy. No randomized trial, however, has ever been performed comparing cardiac transplantation to alternative medical or surgical treatment protocols.

The 1996 annual report of the US Scientific Registry for Organ Transplantation (1) calculated survival of cardiac transplantation patients between October 1987 and December 1994. Actuarial 1-year survival was 82.3% at 1 year and 74.5% at 3 years. UNOS data suggest that 3-year actuarial post–heart transplant survival may be slightly higher among whites (75.4%) than blacks (68.3%) and Hispanics (70.7%). Male recipients have a slightly higher 3-year survival rate (75.2%) than do female recipients (71.8%). The 3-year survival

Table 17.10.   Heart Failure Decompensation: Issues to Address to Obviate the Need for Transplant

- Are there large areas of potentially reversible myocardial ischemia?
- Has new onset of atrial fibrillation or other atrial arrhythmia occurred?
- Is heart block present that might respond to pacemaker insertion?
- Is excessive alcohol consumption a problem?
- Is hyperthyroidism or hypothyroidism present?
- Is poorly controlled diabetes mellitus present?
- Is there excessive afterload (hypertension)?
- Is diuretic prescription appropriately aggressive?
- Are negative inotropic drugs being used?
- Is therapy with nonsteroidal anti-inflammatory agents occurring?
- Is there poor compliance with diet (salt and fluid) and medication prescription?
- Does obesity account for the symptoms?
- Is sleep apnea (particularly obstructive) syndrome present?
- Can cardiovascular deconditioning be improved?
- Is there intercurrent infection present that might respond to antimicrobials?
- Are symptoms actually related to cardiac dysfunction?

for patients aged 1 year or less was 60.4%; and for patients aged 65 years or greater, it was 65.7%.

The Cardiac Transplant Research Database Group (CTRD), a collaborative effort among 30 large U.S. heart transplant centers, representing both academic and community practice programs, analyzed risk factors for death after cardiac transplantation using multivariable parametric risk analysis (6,8,9,18,19). A study of 1719 consecutive primary transplants performed between January 1, 1990, and June 30, 1992, with a mean follow-up of 13.9 months (actuarial survival in this group was 85% at 1 year) demonstrated that independent risk factors for death included younger and older recipient ages, ventilator support at the time of transplantation, higher pulmonary vascular resistance, older donor age, smaller donor body surface area, greater donor requirement for inotropic support, diabetes mellitus in the donor, longer ischemic times (a continuous variable), diffuse donor heart wall motion abnormalities by echocardiography, and for pediatric donors, donor death from causes other than closed head trauma. This analysis demonstrated that the early postoperative mortality (the 30-day mark) was 7% overall, but it increased to 11% when donor age exceeded 50 years, and was 12% when donor inotropic support exceeded 20 μg/kg/min of combined dobutamine and dopamine doses (Table 17.11). The 30-day mortality was 22% when diffuse echocardiographic wall motion abnormalities were detected in the donor heart.

A separate analysis focusing on recipient characteristics demonstrated that the two most common causes of death overall were infection and early graft failure, which accounted for 45% of the deaths. As mentioned, other significant risk factors included ventilator support at the time of transplantation, abnormal renal function, lower pretransplantation cardiac output, and higher pulmonary vascular resistance. The recipient age effect was greatest in patients under 5 years of age (1-year survival rate of 68% in this group versus 85% for all others). Patients aged 60 years and older had a 1-year survival rate of 81%. Transplantation of a blood type O heart into a non-O recipient had a lower 1-year survival rate than did blood type O into a blood type O recipient (82 versus 88%). The adverse effect of a long ischemic time was most notable after 4 h (1-month survival of 71% with ischemic times longer than 4 h versus 85% when less than 4 h). Table 17.11 summarizes both the overall and the 30-day mortality effect of factors found important in this database.

Table 17.11.   Recipient and Donor Risk Factors for Death after Heart Transplantation

Risk Factor	Overall Mortality (Hazard), p value	30-Day Mortality (Logistic), p value
Recipient		
Demographic		
Age		
Younger	.006	.04
Older	.0005	.18
Clinical		
Ventilator at transplant	.00006	.01
Ventricular assist device		.02
Previous sternotomy		.02
Donor		
Demographic		
Adult recipient/donor age older	<.0001	.02
Male recipient/donor female: donor body surface smaller	.003	.01
Clinical		
Ischemic time longer	.0003	.03
Inotropic support increased	.01	.009
Diabetes	.01	.07
If child, cause of death not closed head trauma	.02	.05
If adult, diffuse wall motion abnormalities on ECG	0.6	.003
Cause of death: cardiac arrest		.01

Reprinted with permission from Young JB, Naftel DC, Bourge RC, et al. Matching the heart donor and heart transplant recipient: clues for successful expansion of the donor pull: a multivariable, multi-institutional report. J Heart Lung Transplant 1994;13:353–365.

Concomitant systemic illnesses that may adversely affect post–heart transplant results should be considered contraindications. Individuals with infiltrative or autoimmune diseases, such as amyloidosis, sarcoidosis, and scleroderma, have post–heart transplant outcomes that are much worse than those for the general transplant population. Severe pulmonary disease patients, particularly those with chronic obstructive lung disease associated with chronic bronchitis and markedly reduced forced expiratory volumes are at risk of significant pulmonary infections. Patients with symptomatic peripheral or cerebrovascular disease have a poor outcome, as do those with irreversible renal or hepatic dysfunction. Immunosuppressant agents, in particular cyclosporine, tacrolimus, and azathioprine have associated renal and hepatic toxicity that can be substantive. Active peptic ulcer disease may be worse in the face of chronic corticosteroid administration; and individuals with symptomatic diverticulitis are at risk of bowel perforation with abdominal catastrophe that can be masked by immunosuppressant drugs (particularly steroids).

Some reports suggest that obesity and severe osteoporosis are adverse risk factors for outcome after heart transplantation. Patients are often excluded from listing for morbid obesity, usually defined as a body mass index greater than 30 kg/m². Finally, patient and family noncompliance with therapeutic recommendations, or refusal to follow suggestions regarding diet, weight loss, exercise activity, and general treatment protocols create management dilemmas in the posttransplant patient that lead to adverse outcome.

FUNCTION OF THE CARDIAC ALLOGRAFT

Table 17.12 summarizes some of the factors that affect the function of the transplanted heart. The transplanted heart does not function entirely normally (11,13,16). Even though some cardiac transplant recipients complete astounding exercise challenges, peak exercise tolerance is generally less than expected when heart transplant patients are matched with control patients without cardiac disease. Hemodynamic performance of the heart is related to (a) donor–recipient atrial asynchrony, (b) whether a bicaval or biatrial anastomotic connection was performed, (c) early restrictive physiologic processes related to rejection and ischemic injury, and (d) the volume-expanded state generally seen with congestive heart failure patients entering surgery for cardiac transplantation.

Also, persistently elevated pulmonary artery pressures can be noted for a time after transplant. Ventricular diastolic pressure rises rather substantially during exercise after cardiac transplantation and an overt restrictive hemodynamic pattern has been documented early postoperatively that usually resolves within 4 to 6 weeks; but it can persist in latent fashion much longer. Rejection episodes can also produce a restrictive hemodynamic pattern. An important donor-related issue that affects allograft function is donor to recipient size mismatch. Usually, donors weigh 20 to 40% less than recipients. A significant negative correlation has been identified between

Table 17.12.   Issues Related to Cardiac Allograft Function

Hemodynamics
- Donor–recipient atrial asynchrony
- Bicaval versus biatrial anastomosis
- Early myocardial restrictive physiologic processes
- Late occult myocardial restrictive physiologic processes
- Persistently elevated pulmonary artery pressures (fixed pulmonary hypertension)
- Volume-expanded states

Allograft denervation
- Altered reflex neuroendocrine control of peripheral vasoconstriction and vasodilation
- Altered Na^+/H_2O regulation via vasopressin, renin, angiotensin, aldosterone secretion
- Absence of anginal syndrome during ischemia
- Absent vagus nerve control (rapid heart rate at rest)
- Blunted heart rate increase during exercise
- Loss of diurnal blood pressure fluctuation
- Hypersensitivity to circulating catecholamines
- Exaggerated response to acetylcholine

Altered humoral homeostatic feedback loops
- Atrial natriuretic secretion enhanced
- Elevated circulating catecholamines during exercise
- Increased paracrine peptides (endothelin)
- Increased levels of renin, angiotensin, aldosterone

Myocardial injury/maladaptation
- Organ preservation and recovery injury (acute ischemia)
- Operative complications
- Allograft rejection
- Cardiac allograft vasculopathy
- Hypertensive heart disease
- Ventricular hypertrophy and remodeling

Donor-related issues
- Effect of brain death on cardiac function
- Possibility of cardiac trauma
- Donor–recipient size mismatch
- Age-related diastolic dysfunction
- Preexisting atherosclerosis
- Preexisting ventricular hypertrophy
- Preexisting cardiomyopathy
- Preexisting structural heart disease (atrial septal defect, anomalous coronary artery anatomy)

donor and recipient weight ratio and resting heart rate, right atrial pressure, and pulmonary capillary wedge pressure at 3 months postoperative.

Denervation produces an altered response to exercise. The denervated cardiac allograft generally has a faster resting heart rate (95 to 110 beats/min) than normal and a slower heart rate acceleration during exercise. Afferent and efferent denervation also alters normal neurohumoral homeostasis by impairing renin–angiotensin–aldosterone regulation, changing cardiac diastolic filling parameters, abolishing normal diurnal variation in blood pressure (at least early after transplant), and shifting cardiac pressure volume curves to the right. Higher filling pressures are required, for the most part, to generate reasonable cardiac output. Many drugs used in the transplant patient also affect allograft function. Cyclosporine (CYC), for example, adversely affects renal perfusion and function, leading to substantive hypertension.

The cardiac allograft is a denervated organ that—in the absence of acute rejection, chronic allograft vasculopathy, or substantive hypertension—performs at rest in a similar, but not entirely identical fashion, to the normal heart. Diastolic dysfunction is noted early after cardiac transplantation in virtually every patient; but it gradually disappears, unless rejection reappears or substantive hypertrophy develops.

LONG-TERM MANAGEMENT AND COMPLICATIONS AFTER CARDIAC TRANSPLANTATION

Rejection

Table 17.13 summarizes the significant complications that occur after heart transplantation. Immunosuppressive difficulties can be quite frustrating, and allograft rejection must be anticipated. Traditionally, cardiac rejection has been classified as hyperacute, acute, and chronic. In an attempt to focus on mechanism, cardiac allograft rejection may also be cell mediated or vascular directed. Chronic rejection traditionally refers to the development of cardiac allograft arteriopathy. Cell-mediated rejection generally refers to the T-cell lymphocytic infiltrative process that is staged with endomyocardial

Table 17.13.   Complications Noted after Heart Transplant

Allograft rejection
- Cellular rejection
- Humoral rejection
- Chronic rejection

Infection
- Bacterial
- Viral

    Cytomegalovirus
    Hepatitis
    Herpes virus
    Epstein-Barr virus
    Fungal
        Candida
        Aspergillosis
        Cryptococcus
    Protozoal
        Toxoplasmosis gondii

Allograft arteriopathy

Malignancy
- Kaposi's sarcoma
- Skin cancers
- Solid-organ malignancies
- Posttransplant lymphoproliferative disorder

Immunosuppressive drug-related difficulties
- Nephrotoxicity
- Seizures
- Meningitis (encephalitis)
- Hypertension
- Dyslipidemia
- Osteoporosis
- Obesity
- Cholelithiasis
- Cholestasis
- Pancreatitis
- Hirsutism
- Gingival hyperplasia
- Dysgeusia
- Sinusitis
- Nasal congestion
- Headache
- Tremor
- Peripheral neuropathy
- Aseptic necrosis of joints
- Mood disturbances
- Cataracts
- Hepatotoxicity
- Anemia
- Leukopenia

biopsy. Vascular-directed rejection refers to B-cell antibody–mediated processes and can be characterized by immunohistochemical staining of endomyocardial biopsy samples.

The most commonly used grading scheme for rejection is a scoring system proposed by the International Society for Heart and Lung Transplantation (ISHLT) (20). This standardized endomyocardial biopsy grading system starts with a grade 0, which designates absence of histologic abnormalities in at least three biopsy specimens, and progresses through to grade 4, a very aggressive, diffuse, polymorphous infiltrate associated with vasculitis, hemorrhage, and extensive myocyte necrosis. Grades 3 and 4 generally require augmentation of immunomodulation and are characterized by the term *acute rejection*. Regular biopsy schedules have been developed. Though most intense surveillance usually occurs the first year after cardiac transplantation, surveillance biopsies are usually performed at regular intervals during long-term management of the post–heart transplant patient.

Although several electrocardiographic, echocardiographic, nuclear, and magnetic resonance imaging techniques have been studied, none detects rejection with sufficient sensitivity and specificity to justify replacement of endomyocardial biopsy. These ancillary studies, however, may provide important adjunctive information when designing management schemes. The same can be said for a multitude of monitoring methods, including determining interleukin 2 (IL-2) or soluble IL-2 receptor levels and measuring myocyte necrosis such as troponin and creatinine phosphokinase.

Rejection posttransplant (defined by an event mandating ad hoc augmentation of immunosuppressive therapy) occurs in 50 to 60% of transplant recipients during the first year. The CTRD analysis suggests that 54% of patients had at least one treated rejection episode in that first year postoperative (18). The mean cumulative number of rejection episodes per patient was 0.8 at 3 months, 1.10 at 6 months, and 1.30 at 12 months. Multivariable analysis of this database suggests that younger donor age and female donor gender were independent risk factors for early-appearing rejection. It should be stressed that 40% of patients were free of rejection episodes the first year, but younger recipient age and female donors remain predictive of an earlier onset of rejection.

Infection

Immunocompromised heart transplant recipients experience significant infection (21,22). The incidence of infection in the CTRD analysis was 0.5 per patient during the first year (19). A total of 21% had one and 11% had more than one significant infection. Two peak periods for infection have been identified. In the first 30 days after the operation, nosocomial infections are prominent; *Staphylococcus* species and Gram-negative organisms are the most frequent agents. The second peak occurs 2 to 6 months postoperative with opportunistic organisms such as cytomegalovirus, *Pneumocystis carinii,* and fungi. *Toxoplasmosis* infection generally occurs about 3 months posttransplant.

Risk factors for infection following cardiac transplantation include mechanical ventilation at the time of transplant and use of lymphocytolytic therapy. When a cytomegalovirus-positive donor heart is placed into a cytomegalovirus-negative recipient, risk for infection is increased. Sternal wound infections account for 25% of the deaths caused by infection. Aggressive prophylactic medication protocols used to attenuate infection include ganciclovir infusions early posttransplant to prevent cytomegalovirus, and long-term therapy with co-trimoxazole to prevent *Pneumocystis, Nocardia,* and urinary tract infections. Chronic oral acyclovir is sometimes prescribed for several months posttransplant in an adjunctive attempt to prevent cytomegalovirus infections.

Aggressive evaluation of all febrile patients includes gastrointestinal endoscopy to isolate cytomegalovirus from the gastrointestinal tract in certain cases, lumbar puncture to exclude central nervous system cryptococcus or aspergillosis and early bronchoscopy to obtain pulmonary secretions and tissue to evaluate cough or radiographic infiltration. Opportunistic infections frequently occur in unusual locations, such as the central nervous system, bone marrow, and gallbladder. Cooperation with pulmonologic, gastroenterologic, hepatologic, and infectious disease experts skilled in the management of immunocompromised patients and access to sophisticated microbiology and pathology laboratories are essential.

Endocarditis Prophylaxis

Infective endocarditis is a rare complication after cardiac transplantation, but it is recommended that immunocompromised cardiac transplant recipients be given antibiotic prophylaxis before procedures that might precipitate bacteremia. According to the American Heart Association and the American Dental Association, an oral protocol for lower risk procedures on patients includes amoxicillin, 3 g orally 1 h before the procedure and 1.5 g 6 h after the initial dose. For allergic patients, erythromycin, 1 g orally 2 h before the procedure then one-half of the initial dose 6 h later is recommended. Although erythromycin increases CYC levels when taken chronically, single doses are not problematic. An alternative is clindamycin given 300 mg orally 1 h before the procedure and 150 mg 6 h after the initial dose.

Prophylactic Vaccination

Another common question arising during long-term post–heart transplant recipient follow-up is what to do about prophylactic vaccination against specific infections (16). Commonly accepted vaccination protocols for solid-organ transplant recipients in general are not yet well characterized. There is concern that use of live virus vaccines in the immunocompromised transplant recipient could produce infection. Another concerning observation has been that some patients seem to have rejection episodes triggered postvaccination. Theoretically the up-regulation of the immune system that occurs after vaccination may in some way increase risk of allograft rejection. These observations have, however, been sporadic and ill-characterized.

Heart transplant candidates should be evaluated for immunity to hepatitis B, measles, mumps, rubella, poliomyelitis, and varicella before transplantation surgery. Individuals not demonstrating immunity could be vaccinated during the pretransplant period, avoiding live virus vaccinations within 3 months of anticipated transplant. In addition, transplant candidates should receive pneumococcal vaccine once and a tetanus diphtheria booster every decade. In the posttransplant period, pneumococcal vaccine boosters should be repeated every 5 or 6 years and tetanus boosters again every decade. Prophylactic high antibody immunoglobulin therapy has been recommended when exposure of nonimmunized heart transplant recipients occurs to tetanus, measles, varicella, or hepatitis B virus. Exposure to influenza A virus can be treated with amantadine and patients developing a rash after varicella exposure should receive high dose acyclovir. The annual influenza vaccination for heart transplant recipients is controversial, but many centers routinely administer influenza vaccine every fall to their transplant recipient population.

Allograft Arteriopathy

Chronic rejection refers to a specific type of coronary artery disease that develops in the transplanted heart (21–24). Allograft arteriopathy appears to be the leading cause of death beyond the first year. Though annual coronary arteriography has been traditionally used to diagnose the problem, intravascular ultrasonography and angioscopy have shown vastly better sensitivity.

Allograft arteriopathy is a proliferative response to endothelial injury. The vascular endothelial surface is a target for cell- and antibody-mediated inflammation, accelerated by dyslipidemia, hypertension, and cytomegalovirus infections common after heart transplant. Alloimmune responses directed toward the endothelium produce endothelial activation, which results in the synthesis of growth factors that, in turn, promote smooth-muscle cell proliferation. Treatment generally centers on intensification of immunotherapy and control of the traditional risk factors for atherosclerosis, such as hypertension and dyslipidemia. Early reports have suggested that diltiazem (25) and pravastatin (26) may have protective effects. The newer immunosuppressive agents rapamycin and mycophenolate may also be more effective in inhibiting smooth-muscle cell proliferation and migration (27–30). Other agents, such as low molecular weight heparin and angiopeptin, are being evaluated (30). A repeat cardiac transplantation is associated with only 50% 1-year survival.

Malignancy

As Table 17.13 indicates, several different malignancies can occur in the heart transplant recipient (16,19,21,31), as with other solid-organ transplantation. The most common are localized skin cancers; squamous cell carcinoma of the skin, however, can be quite problematic. Carcinoma of the lung, gastrointestinal tract, breast, and prostate all require surveillance. Posttransplant lymphoproliferative disorder (PTLD), a non-Hodgkin's type of lymphoma, is generally

B-cell in origin; and some posttransplant lymphoproliferative disorders have regressed with only a reduction of immunosuppression. Epstein-Barr virus may play a role in these malignancies, since nuclear and membrane proteins characteristic of this virus have been identified using molecular techniques in these B-cell proliferations.

Treatment of posttransplant malignancy is difficult. A variety of cancer chemotherapy and radiation protocols are undergoing evaluation but definitive and specific recommendations cannot be made now.

Hypertension

Hypertension after heart transplant has been related to immunosuppressive drugs (16,21,22,32). Cyclosporine is particularly culpable; however, chronic steroid administration also contributes to the problem. Note that compared to cardiac allograft recipients, liver transplant patients on similar CYC doses have less blood pressure elevation. Denervation of the heart contributes to hypertension as well. Treatment of hypertension post–heart transplant is largely empiric. Calcium channel blockers, angiotensin-converting enzyme inhibitors, β-blockers, central and peripheral α-blockers, diuretics, and direct-acting vasodilators have all been used alone or in varying combinations.

Diltiazem not only acts as an antihypertensive agent but also substantially decreases cyclosporine requirements by increasing drug levels. High doses of angiotensin-converting enzyme inhibitors or angiotensin II receptor blocking agents are necessary because of the excess of circulating renin levels in transplant patients; if these drugs are chosen, one should carefully observe renal function parameters, including potassium levels. β-Blockers are difficult to use in the heart transplant population because of allograft denervation. β-Blockers attenuate the heart rate increase response to exercise and can precipitate unacceptable bradyarrhythmia or heart block. The use of rate-responsive atrial pacemakers allows more effective use of β-blockers post–heart transplant. Obviously, dietary control of salt consumption and aerobic exercise prescription must always be components of hypertension management of the post–heart transplant patient.

Seizures

Grand mal seizures have been seen with some frequency during administration of cytolytic therapy, particularly OKT3 (16,21,22) or with CYC. These seizures generally occur in the first several weeks after surgery, but can occasionally manifest later in the first year. Of course, heart transplant recipients are at risk of having any type of seizure disorder. When evaluating patients presenting with a grand mal seizure posttransplant, one should consider drug toxicities as the cause for the disorder and should use drugs cautiously, since many seizure-control preparations alter cyclosporine levels (e.g., dilantin, phenobarbital, and carbamazepine all decrease CYC blood levels).

Nephrotoxicity

Deterioration of renal function post–heart transplant occurs commonly. Many heart failure patients have some renal insufficiency preoperatively, and many drugs administered after transplant, such as cyclosporine and tacrolimus, adversely affect renal function (32–34). Renal histopathologic studies may demonstrate substantive glomerular sclerosis. Adequate renal function is imperative before subjecting a patient to transplant, and efforts should be made to avoid drugs that are concomitantly nephrotoxic, if at all possible. Common offenders include nonsteroidal anti-inflammatory agents, antibiotics, certain gastrointestinal preparations, and high doses of immunosuppressants.

Dyslipidemia

Most patients develop lipid abnormalities after cardiac transplantation (21,22,35,36). The guidelines for lipid-lowering therapy in nontransplant dyslipidemic populations do not necessarily address the specific treatment needs of the cardiac transplant recipient. Indeed, lipid-lowering agents in the heart transplant recipient carry significant risk. Rhabdomyolysis occurring in patients on higher doses of 3-hydroxy-3-methylglutaryl coenzyme A (HmG CoA) inhibitors in the face of cyclosporine therapy is well characterized. When low doses of lovastatin, simvastatin, or pravastatin have been used, however, the incidence of rhabdomyolysis seems less. Note that one prospective, randomized, but unblinded single-center clinical trial suggests that development of allograft arteriopathy and survival improved with the routine use of pravastatin in the early postoperative period (26,37). Pravastatin may have immunosuppressive and smooth-muscle antimitotic effects in addition to its lipid-lowering action.

Other Immunosuppressive Drug-Related Difficulties

Osteoporosis, which leads to compression fractures, degenerative joint disease, and aseptic necrosis of the femoral heads (38), is primarily related to the use of steroids. Obesity poses a significant problem posttransplant, and patients on steroids are challenged to lose weight. Cholelithiasis occurs with increased frequency in individuals on CYC, and any abdominal discomfort requires attention to the gallbladder (39). Pancreatitis can be caused by cyclosporine as well as azathioprine. Hirsutism and gingival hyperplasia are particularly troublesome complications of cyclosporine. Sometimes switching from cyclosporine to tacrolimus or vice versa, helps control these nuisance side effects. Other frustrating difficulties include hyperkalemia, hypomagnesemia, and hyperuricemia induced by CYC.

Gout can be particularly problematic with most patients on azathioprine, since allopurinol is relatively contraindicated and nonsteroidal anti-inflammatory agents worsen renal function in this setting. Gout is best treated acutely with colchicine or pulses of high-dose prednisone. If allopurinol is required, consider switching from azathioprine to mycophenolate mofetil for immunosuppression.

Troublesome paresthesias, insomnia, anxiety, dysgeusia, rhinorrhea, sinusitis, nasal congestion, and headache seem to be associated with cyclosporin and sometimes improve after switching to tacrolimus.

IMMUNOSUPPRESSIVE AGENTS IN OVERVIEW

Though modulation of immunosuppressive therapies in the post–heart transplant recipient is best done by the transplant cardiologist responsible for caring for the patient, a general understanding of these drugs, particularly with reference to toxicity and modulation of their effects by concomitant drug therapies is important. Table 17.14 summarizes selected points about the most frequently used immunosuppressive agents after cardiac transplantation. Table 17.15 focuses on drugs that are frequently used in the heart failure, hypertensive, or dyslipidemic patient that might affect cyclosporine levels.

SUMMARY

Cardiac transplantation substantially attenuates the devastating morbidity and mortality of advanced heart failure. Proper patient

Table 17.14.   Selected Characteristics of Immunosuppressive Agents

Drug	Mechanism	Toxicity	Increases [CYC]	Decreases [CYC]
Cyclosporine	IL-2 signal transduction blocked	HTN Nephrotoxicity Neurotoxicity (seizures, tremor, paresthesias) Hirsutism Gingival hyperplasia Dysgeusia	Erythromycin Ketoconazole Diltiazem Cimetidine Ciprofloxacin Grapefruit juice	Dilantin Phenobarbital Rifampin Cholestyramine Tegretol
Steroids	Lymphocytolytic Alters B-cell antigenic response	Glucose intolerance HTN Osteoporosis Cataracts Growth retardation		
Azathioprine	Purine antimetabolite	Leukopenia Pancreatitis Stomatitis Cholestatic jaundice Macrocytic anemia (Allopurinol potentiates; azathioprine effects toxicity)		
Methotrexate	Folate analog Purine antimetabolite	Leukopenia Hepatitis Stomatitis		
Tacrolimus	IL-2 signal transduction blocked	HTN Nephrotoxicity Neurotoxicity Glucose intolerance		
Mycophenolate mofetil	Inhibits purine synthesis	GI (nausea, vomiting, diarrhea)		
Cytolytic agents (OKT3, antilymphocyte, and thymocyte globulin)	Lymphocyte depletion Pulmonary edema Seizures	Fever Meningitis		

HTN, hypertension; *GI*, gastrointestinal.

Table 17.15. Drugs Frequently Used in the Heart Failure, Hypertensive, or Dyslipidemia Patients That Might Affect Cyclosporin Levels or Other Aspects of the Posttransplant Milieu

Drug	Putative Effects	Mechanism
Acetazolamide	↑ [CYC]	↑ CYC absorption ↓ CYC metabolism Altered CYC distribution
Cholestyramine	↓ [CYC]	Altered CYC absorption
Diltiazem	↑ [CYC) Worse gingival hyperplasia Renal protective	↓ CYC metabolism
Disopyramide	↓ Serum creatinine	Unknown
Enalapril	Renal protective	Unknown
Felodipine	Renal protective Worse gingival hyperplasia	Unknown
Furosemide	Increased nephrotoxicity	↓ [Na⁺] ↓ Intravascular volume
HmG CoA reduction inhibitors	Myositis Rhabdomyolysis with nephrotoxicity	Decreased statin metabolism
Mannitol	Increased nephrotoxicity	Unknown
Metolazone	Renal protective	Unknown
Nicardipine	↑ [CYC] Worse gingival hyperplasia Renal protective	↓ CYC metabolism
Nifedipine	Worse gingival hyperplasia	Unknown
Nitrendipine	Worse gingival hyperplasia	Unknown
Prazosin	Renal protective	↑ Renal blood flow
Propranolol	Antagonistic immunosuppressive effect	Unknown
Spironolactone	Renal protective	Unknown
Verapamil	↑ [CYC] Worse gingival hyperplasia Renal protective	↓ CYC metabolism
Warfarin	↓ [CYC] ↑ Prothombin activity	↑ CYC metabolism

selection, aggressive pretransplant management of heart failure, reasonable donor selection and care, and compulsive postoperative surveillance with both prophylactic and ad hoc treatment protocols are essential to satisfactory outcomes. Common sense and close communication between the transplant center and primary caregivers will ensure that these complex patients have the greatest chance for long-term success.

REFERENCES

1. Annual report of the U.S. Scientific Registry of Transplant Recipients and the Organ Procurement and Transplantation Network—transplant data: 1988–1996. Bethesda, MD: US Department of Health and Human Services, 1997.
2. Evans RW, Manninen DL, Dong FB. The National Heart Transplantation Study: final report. Seattle: Battelle Human Affairs Research Centers, 1991.
3. Evans RW, Manninen DL, Garrison LP Jr, et al. Donor availability as the primary determinant of the future of heart transplant. JAMA 1986;255:1892.
4. Evans RW. Socioeconomic aspects of heart transplantation. Curr Opin Cardiol 1995;10(2):169–179.
5. Hosenpud JD, Breen TJ, Edwards EB, et al. The effect of transplant center volume on cardiac transplant outcome. JAMA 1994;271(23):1844–1849.
6. Jarcho J, Naftel DC, Shroyer TW, et al. Influence of HLA mismatch on rejection after heart transplantation: a multi-institutional study. J Heart Lung Transplant 1964;13:583–596.
7. Sweeny MS, Lammermeier DE, Frazier OH, et al. Extension of donor criteria in cardiac transplantation: surgical risk versus supply side economics. Ann Thorac Surg 1990;50:7–15.
8. Baldwin JC, Anderson JL, Boucek MM, et al. Task Force 2 (Bethesda conference—cardiac transplantation): donor guidelines. J Am Coll Cardiol 1993;22:15.
9. Young JB, Naftel DC, Bourge RC, et al. Matching the heart donor and heart transplant recipient: clues for successful expansion of the donor pull: a multivariable, multi-institutional report. J Heart Lung Transplant 1994;13:353–365.
10. Stevenson LW, Miller LW. Cardiac transplantation as therapy for heart failure. Curr Probl Cardiol 1991;16:219–305.
11. Young JB, Winters WL Jr, Bourge R, et al. Task Force 4 (Bethesda conference—heart transplantation): function of the heart transplant recipient. J Am Coll Cardiol 1993;22:31.
12. Bourge RC, Naftel DC, Costanzo-Nordin MR, et al. Pretransplantation risk factors for death after heart transplantation: a multi-institutional study. J Heart Lung Transplant 1993;12:549.
13. Costanzo MR, Augustine S, Bourge R, et al. Selection and treatment of candidates for heart transplantation. A statement for health professionals from the Committee on Heart Failure and Cardiac Transplantation of the Council on Clinical Cardiology, American Heart Association. Circulation 1995;92:3593–3612.
14. Francis GS. Determinants of prognosis in patients with heart failure. J Heart Lung Transplant 1994;13:5113–5116.
15. Miller LW, Kubo SH, Young JB, et al. Report of the Consensus Conference on candidate selection for cardiac transplantation. J Heart Lung Transplant 1995;14:562–571.
16. O'Connell JB, Bourge RC, Costanzo-Nordin MR, et al. Cardiac transplantation: recipient selection, donor procurement, and medical follow-up. A statement for health professionals from the Committee on Cardiac Transplantation of the

Council on Clinical Cardiology, American Heart Association. Circulation 1992; 86:1061–1079.

17. Mudge GH, Goldstein S, Addonizio LJ, et al. Twenty-fourth Bethesda conference: cardiac transplantation: Task Force 3: recipient guidelines/prioritization. J Am Coll Cardiol 1993;22:21–31.

18. Kobashigawa JA, Kirklin JK, Naftel DC, et al. Pretransplantation risk factors for acute rejection after heart transplantation: a multi-institutional study. J Heart Lung Transplant 1993;12:355–366.

19. Miller LW, Naftel DC, Bourge RC, et al. Infection following cardiac transplantation: a multi-institutional analysis. Transplant Cardiologists' Research Database Group. J Heart Lung Transplant 1992;11-I(Part 2):192.

20. Billingham ME, Cary NR, Hammond EH, et al. A working foundation for the standardization of nomenclature in the diagnosis of heart and lung rejection. Heart Rejection Study Group. J Heart Transplant 1990;9:587.

21. Miller LW. Long-term complications of cardiac transplantation. Prog Cardiovasc Dis 1991;32:229.

22. Miller LW, Schlant RC, Kosbashigawa J, et al. Task Force 5 (Bethesda conference–cardiac transplantation): complications. J Am Coll Cardiol 1993;22:41.

23. Miller LW, Wolford TL, Donohue TJ, et al. Cardiac allograft vasculopathy: new insights from intravascular ultrasound and coronary flow measurements. Transplant Rev 1995;9:77–96.

24. Johnson DE, Gao SZ, Schroeder JS, et al. The spectrum of coronary artery pathologic findings in human cardiac allografts. J Heart Transplant 1989;8:349.

25. Klintmalm GB, Ascher NL, Busuttil RW, et al. RS-61443 for treatment-resistant human liver rejection. Transplant Proc 1993;25:697.

26. Kobashigawa JA, Katznelson S, Laks H, et al. Effect of pravastatin on outcomes after cardiac transplantation. N Engl J Med 1995;333:621.

27. Ensley RD, Bristow MR, Olsen SL, et al. The use of mycophenolate mofetil (RS-61443) in human heart transplant recipients. Transplantation 1993;56:75–82.

28. Kirklin JK, Bourge RC, Naftel DC, et al. Treatment of recurrent heart rejection with mycophenolate mofetil (RS-61443): initial clinical experience. J Heart Lung Transplant 1994;13:444–450.

29. Taylor DO, Ensley RD, Olsen SL, et al. Mycophenolate mofetil (RS-61443): preclinical, clinical and three-year experience in heart transplantation. J Heart Lung Transplant 1994;13:571–582.

30. Costanzo-Nordin MR, Cooper DKC, Jessup M, et al. Task Force 6 (Bethesda conference—cardiac transplantation): future developments. J Am Coll Cardiol 1993;22–54.

31. Penn I. Cancers after cyclosporine therapy. Transplant Proc 1988;20:276–279.

32. Kahan BD. Cyclosporine. N Engl J Med 1989;321:1725–1738.

33. Thomson AW. FK-506: profile of an important new immunosuppressant. Transplantation Rev 1990;4:1–13.

34. Pham SM, Kormos RL, Hattler BG, et al. A prospective trial of tacrolimus (FK506) in clinical heart transplantation: intermediate-term results. J Thorac Cardiovasc Surg 1996;111:764–772.

35. Ballantyne CM, Podet EJ, Patsch WP, et al. Effects of cyclosporine therapy on plasma lipoprotein levels. JAMA 1989;26:53.

36. Ballantyne CM, Radovancevic B, Farmer JA, et al. Hyperlipidemia after heart transplantation: report of a 6-year experience with treatment recommendations. J Am Coll Cardiol 1992;19:1315.

37. Vaughan CJ, Murphy MB. Statins do more than just lower cholesterol. Lancet 1996;348:1079–1082.

38. Rich GM, Mudge GH, Laffel GL, et al. Cyclosporine A and prednisone associated osteoporosis in heart transplant recipients. J Heart Lung Transplant 1992;11: 940–948.

39. Merrell SW, Ames SA, Nelson EW, et al. Major abdominal complications following cardiac transplantation. Arch Surg 1989;124:889–894.

Section 4

Summary and Future Trends in Heart Failure

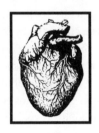

Chapter 18

Future Trends in Heart Failure
Greater Insight into Pathophysiologic Processes, Diagnosis,
and Treatment

Roger M. Mills Jr. and James B. Young

As discussed in preceding chapters, heart failure is now a true pandemic, accounting for extraordinary morbidity and mortality. We have emphasized evidence-based team medical practice, with reliance on physician extenders integrating multidisciplinary approaches to heart failure patient care, and interdependence between medical and surgical approaches to the syndrome. Unfortunately, in the United States the large cohort of Baby Boomers is now moving into the stage of life at which an increased incidence of heart failure is expected. Furthermore, worldwide epidemiologic processes in cardiovascular disease suggest that the global burden of heart failure will only grow. Fortunately growing expertise in other countries makes important discoveries with respect to heart failure therapeutics more likely. With the immediacy of electronic communication systems, new medical technologies will rapidly disseminate throughout the world. Volume-reduction surgery for dilated cardiomyopathy, for example, was first performed in Brazil and subsequently rapidly moved into clinical trials in the United States.

The organization of medicine will continue its rapid social evolution. Economic issues will obviously drive decision making, but they will likely become aligned with patient-driven demands as payers' perspectives broaden to include the consideration of optimal treatment outcomes. With this trend, the physician's role will evolve to a less hands-on approach with more team leader responsibilities. The multidisciplinary team will include clinical nurse specialists, exercise physiologists, dietitians, and pharmacists. Patients will take increased responsibility for self-care by making major changes in lifestyle and monitoring their own physiologic parameters.

The pharmaceutical industry will likely support comprehensive disease management programs based on clinical trials evidence. Clinical trials will include socioeconomic analysis of the various treatment regimens being evaluated to allow determination of cost-effective approaches to heart failure. Tremendous emphasis will be placed on primary and secondary prevention of cardiac disease and subsequent heart failure. Early detection of hypertension and lipid abnormalities will allow earlier treatment with, ultimately, a reduction in the prevalence of heart failure. Secondary prevention and delay of progression of ventricular dysfunction will also be stressed; these tactics will become indicators of quality and value in new health care organizational structures.

Likely future scientific advances were summarized in a report by the National Heart, Lung, and Blood Institute (NHLBI) (1,2). The Panel on Heart Failure Research recommended four specific areas for support by the National Institutes of Health to better understand and more effectively treat the problem of heart failure. An improved national network of clinicians and scientists should be created to interact intimately with respect to determining causes of heart failure and to developing subsequent practical and effective solutions. Emphasis was placed on supporting promising basic science approaches, such as gene manipulation therapies, to interdict development of ventricular dysfunction and subsequent clinical heart failure syndromes. Newer basic research techniques could supplement existing ones in exploiting ongoing molecular genetic research, setting the stage for heart failure research in the next century. Particular emphasis was placed on supporting research that would link information being generated by the Human Genome Project (HGP) to insight being gained into myocyte growth and hypertrophy. Theoretically, this information would allow futuristic gene transfer technology to focus on the problem of remodeling associated with heart failure. Finally, the panel stressed the importance of attracting and retaining clinicians and scientists to study heart failure in a global context.

Table 18.1 lists specific heart failure research agendas suggested by the NHLBI panel. Studies designed to understand and regulate cardiac apoptosis were believed essential, because the loss of appropriately functioning cardiac myocytes seems to be the fundamental difficulty in initiating and subsequently aggravating ventricular dysfunction in clinical heart failure. Differentiating between necrosis

Table 18.1.   Areas of Future Heart Failure Research

Perform studies designed to understand and regulate cardiac apoptosis
Characterize better the cardiac cell cycle and determine how to control cell
 proliferation and growth
Study the integrated physiologic, molecular, biochemical, and multiorgan factors
 important in heart failure's global milieu
Develop better animal models of heart failure
Determine the contribution of myocyte energy depletion to heart failure
Understand the factors leading to fatal arrhythmias in heart failure
Determine the ability of pharmacologic agents or mechanical left ventricular assist
 devices to induce regression of heart failure abnormalities (particularly
 remodeling)
Describe more accurately the morphometric and functional alterations of intact
 failing hearts
Link therapeutic insight developed from pathophysiologic studies to clinical trials
 so that evidence-based treatment strategies can be developed

Data from Cohn JN, Bristow MR, Chien KR, et al. Report of the National Heart, Lung, and Blood Institute Special Emphasis Panel on Heart Failure Research. Circulation 1997;95:766–770; and Lenfant C. Fixing the failing heart. Circulation 1997;95:771–772.

and apoptosis is important, since apoptosis appears to be mediated by multiple factors that create a cycle of programmed cell death distinct from the sudden necrosis occurring after a major ischemic event. Blocking apoptotic signaling pathways might halt heart failure progression. Adult myocytes are terminally differentiated and incapable of regeneration. Restoration of their proliferative capacity could foster a proliferation of new cells and true healing of the heart.

Future studies will focus on the physiological, molecular, biochemical, and peripheral organ interactions that account for clinical heart failure. As the Panel on Heart Failure Research pointed out, simply focusing on the myocyte or left ventricle alone in heart failure overlooks important interactions that occur in the syndrome and that contribute to a variety of signaling abnormalities that perpetuate the condition. For example, the hemodynamic overload characteristic of heart failure is associated with disturbances of myocardial signaling mechanisms that up regulate expression of growth factors, cytokines, other inflammatory proteins, and nitric oxide. These factors affect the phenotypic expression of myocytes, fibroblasts, vascular smooth muscle cells, and endothelial cells, which constitute the remodeling phenomenon.

Multiorgan autocrine and paracrine feedback loops must be better characterized, so that specific pharmacotherapeutic targets can be developed. To study these issues, new technologies and improved animal models of heart failure will be needed. Large animal models of heart failure should have phases of compensation and decompensation, and remodeling should be characterized by ventricular hypertrophy and chamber dilation similar to that seen in the clinical world.

Future research will clarify the contribution of energy depletion to the heart failure syndrome. Energy stores are not necessarily depleted in failing myocytes, but limitations in energy transfer are present. At the molecular level, physical limitations in energy substrate availability because of obstructive coronary artery disease and ventricular hypertrophy–mediated alterations in subendocardial capillary perfusion must be better understood before they can be addressed effectively.

Fatal arrhythmias seen in patients with ventricular dysfunction may reflect mutant genes mediating structurally and functionally abnormal potassium and sodium channels. By more specifically identifying the ion channels associated with perturbed signaling pathways, better approaches to antiarrhythmic therapy in this high-risk population can be anticipated. Alternative measures will include vastly more sophisticated arrhythmia detection and termination machinery implanted in heart failure patients at high risk for arrhythmogenic death.

Future practitioners will see pharmacologic techniques to induce regression of ventricular remodeling (hypertrophy and dilation). Improved use of existing drugs and unique new agents will expand with angiotensin-converting enzyme inhibitors being coupled to other drugs, such as β-adrenergic blockers and specific angiotensin II receptor site blockers in more aggressive fashion. The role of calcium channel blocking agents will be clarified, and new intravenous agents will be combined with more aggressive inpatient management of heart failure, which may include earlier and more widespread insertion of left ventricular assist devices.

Cardiac transplantation will remain limited by insufficient donor organs; however, implantation of left ventricular assist devices as an alternative to cardiac transplantation or as a bridge to recovery will likely occur. Preliminary data suggest recovery in patients treated early (presumably before irretrievable apoptosis has begun) with ventricular assist device insertion. Clinical trials of these innovative machines will be required.

Better understanding of the structural and functional alterations of failing hearts will occur with studies that define specific gene expression leading to myocyte and fibroblast growth and remodeling. Specifically, the roles of hemodynamic factors, growth hormones, cytokines, and yet to be clarified or discovered paracrine mechanisms will be elucidated, and the capacity of the myocardium to reverse detrimental remodeling will be defined.

Finally, the future will see clinical trials designed to test both medical and surgical therapeutic concepts in heart failure. Results from these trials will provide the support for new and more effective treatment algorithms in heart failure.

SUMMARY

Emerging lines of research will provide new targets for intense, evidence-based heart failure treatment and better understanding of methods to prevent heart failure. We have offered an overview of the state-of-the-art approach to heart failure patients. By encompassing the problem from pathophysiologic insight to social issues, we hope to improve treatment for this devastating epidemic. We are enthusiastic and optimistic.

REFERENCES
1. Cohn JN, Bristow MR, Chien KR, et al. Report of the National Heart, Lung, and Blood Institute Special Emphasis Panel on Heart Failure Research. Circulation 1997;95:766–770.
2. Lenfant C. Fixing the failing heart. Circulation 1997;95:771–772.

Appendix

Model Management Strategies in Heart Failure

Santosh G. Menon

Appendix I: *(See the following page.)* Clinical laboratory evaluation of a patient with new onset heart failure. **Notes:** *(a)* Most common ECG finding in a patient with CHF is nonspecific ST/T changes. Presence of Q waves, loss of R wave, and persistent ST segment elevation suggesting an left ventricular aneurysm point CAD as the cause of CHF. Chest x-ray usually shows cardiomegaly and pulmonary congestion in > 90% of patients with CHF. Hematocrits < 25 can produce signs and symptoms of CHF, even in patients with no underlying cardiac disease. If serum creatinine is elevated, consider renal failure as the cause of fluid overload. Hypothyroidism and hyperthyroidism may cause or aggravate CHF. *(b)* ECG is a valuable tool in patients with CHF; it helps exclude valvular heart disease and mechanical defects (VSD, LV aneurysm) and confirms the presence of dilated cardiomyopathy. Typical findings include dilation of the LV, increased end-systolic and end-diastolic dimensions, and reduced fractional shortening and EF. Radionuclide ventriculography gives a more accurate estimation of EF and a better assessment of right ventricular function. *(c)* Defects may be caused by acute ischemia (stunned myocardium) or chronic severe ischemia (hibernating myocardium). Patients with fixed perfusions defects at 4 h should undergo reinjection and scanning at 24 h to assess viability of myocardium in poorly perfused areas. *(d)* Sarcoidosis, amyloidosis, acute myocarditis, allergic granulomatosis, hemochromatosis, and doxorubicin cardiomyopathy. *JVD,* jugular venous distension; *DOE,* dyspnea on exertion; *PND,* paroxysmal nocturnal dyspnea; *CHF,* congestive heart failure; *COPD,* chronic obstructive lung disease; *CXR,* chest x-ray; *CBC,* complete blood count; *TSH,* thyroid-stimulating hormone; *EF,* ejection fraction; *PET,* positron-emission tomography; *LV,* left ventricular; *MUGA,* multi-gated acquisition.

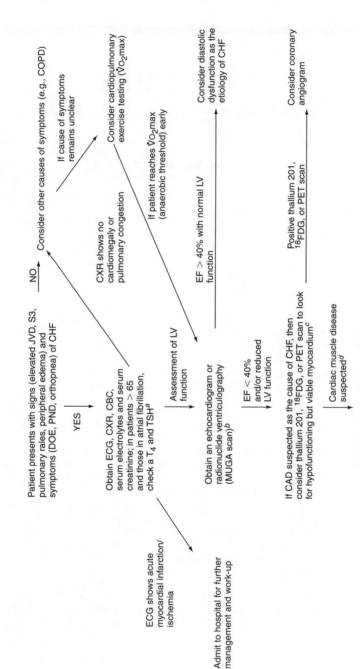

Patient presents with signs (elevated JVD, S3, pulmonary rales, peripheral edema) and symptoms (DOE, PND, orthopnea) of CHF

YES

Obtain ECG, CXR, CBC, serum electrolytes and serum creatinine; in patients > 65 and those in atrial fibrillation, check a T_4 and TSH[a]

ECG shows acute myocardial infarction/ischemia

Admit to hospital for further management and work-up

Assessment of LV function

Obtain an echocardiogram or radionuclide ventriculography (MUGA scan)[b]

EF < 40% and/or reduced LV function

EF > 40% with normal LV function

If CAD suspected as the cause of CHF, then consider thallium 201, [18]FDG, or PET scan to look for hypofunctioning but viable myocardium[c]

Cardiac muscle disease suspected[d]

Consider an endomyocardial biopsy (if clinically indicated)

Positive thallium 201, [18]FDG, or PET scan

Consider coronary angiogram

Consider diastolic dysfunction as the etiology of CHF

NO

Consider other causes of symptoms (e.g., COPD)

CXR shows no cardiomegaly or pulmonary congestion

If cause of symptoms remains unclear

Consider cardiopulmonary exercise testing ($\dot{V}O_2$max)

If patient reaches $\dot{V}O_2$max (anaerobic threshold) early

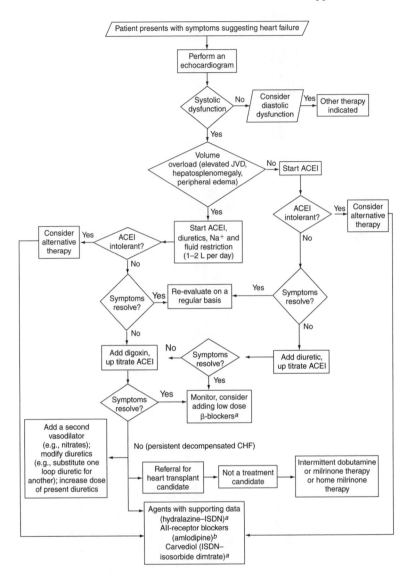

Appendix II: Outpatient management of the heart failure patient. **Notes:** *(a)* For example, carvedilol 3.125 mg PO bid; titrate up after 2 weeks if patient is tolerating it. *(b)* Losartan. *ACEI*, angiotensin-converting enzyme inhibitor; *JVD*, jugular venous distension.

Patient with heart failure refractory to medical management. Gather the following clinical data:

1. Age of patient
2. ABO blood type
3. History of blood transfusions
4. History of any co-morbid conditions, e.g., insulin-dependent diabetes mellitus, intrinsic lung disease, renal disease, morbid obesity, tobacco abuse, malignancy, noncompliance, drug or alcohol addiction, psychiatric problems, risk factors for HIV or viral hepatitis
5. PFTs with DLCO
6. Presence of malignancy
7. Echocardiogram/radionuclide ventriculography
8. Right and left heart catheterization results
9. $\dot{V}O_2$ max
10. Carotid duplex examination
11. Segmental peripheral Dopplers
12. Clearance with insurance company

Could heart failure respond to conventional surgery, e.g., revascularization, valve replacement, or aneurysectomy

or

Could symptoms of heart failure respond to intensification of medical management, e.g., increasing dose of diuretics or ACEI

Yes, intensify medical regimen and defer transplantation temporarily; reassess periodically

Yes; proceed with surgery with transplant as a back up (if no contraindications present)

No; would the benefit of cardiac transplantation justify the risk as assessed by an experienced cardiac transplant team

Yes; list for cardiac transplant; consider bridging devices

No; consider home inotropic therapy, hospice, and other palliative measures

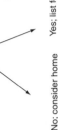

Notes

1. Traditionally 60 years of age has been the upper age limit for consideration for cardiac transplantation at most centers. Patients > 65 years may be considered at some centers.

2. Patients with O blood type typically have a longer waiting period for cardiac transplantation.

3. Patients who received blood transfusions may be sensitized to foreign antigens and may require a prospective cross-match with the donor heart.

4. Patients with IDDM with end-organ damage (e.g., retinopathy, nephropathy, or peripheral neuropathy); moderate to severe COPD (FVC < 50% or FEV1.0 < 1 L); ongoing tobacco, drug, or alcohol abuse; or significant psychiatric problems that may interfere with the patient's ability to comply with the intense postoperative regimen are usually not candidates for cardiac transplantation. Body weight > 30% of ideal is considered a relative contraindication. Patients who are HIV positive or hepatitis C positive are not candidates for cardiac transplantation at most centers.

5. Presence of a uncured malignancy is a contraindication to cardiac transplantation.

6. Patients with an ejection fraction of < 20% are at a higher risk for death from heart failure (1).

7. Excessive elevation of PVR or transpulmonary gradient (PVR > 4–6 Wood units or a TPG > 15 mm Hg that is fixed) makes the patient unacceptable for cardiac transplantation (2).

8. Peak exercise oxygen consumption measured during maximal exercise ($\dot{V}O_2$max) provides a measurement of cardiovascular reserve and helps differentiate CHF from pulmonary disease. Patients with $\dot{V}O_2$max < 14 mL/kg/min should be listed for cardiac transplantation.

9. Patients > 40 years should have carotid Doppler study to assess the patency of the carotid arteries. Carotid endarterectomy may be performed before heart transplantation to minimize the risk of postoperative cerebrovascular events (3).

10. Should be done on patients with a history of claudication. Correctable lesion, should be fixed before transplantation.

11. Most government and third-party carriers pay for cardiac transplantation. A review of finances should be done before accepting a patient for cardiac transplantation, since the cost of transplantation, medication, etc. can be tremendous.

Appendix III: Information needed for cardiac transplant evaluation. *ACEI*, angiotensin-converting enzyme inhibitor; *PFTs*, pulmonary function tests; *DLCO*, diffusion capacity; *TPG*, transpulmonary gradient; *FVC*, forced vital capacity; *FEV 1.0*, forced expiratory volume in 1 s.

REFERENCES
1. Keogh AM, Baron DW, Hickie JB. Prognostic guides in patients with idiopathic or ischemic dilated cardiomyopathy assessed for cardiac transplantation. Am J Cardiol 1990;65:903–908.
2. O'Connell JB, Bourge RC, Costanzo-Nordin MR, et al. Cardiac transplantation: recipient selection, donor procurement, and medical follow-up. Circulation 1992;86:1061–1079.
3. Costanzo MR, Augustine SA, Bourge R, et al. Selection and treatment of candidates for heart transplantation. Circulation 1995;95:3593–3612.

Index

More Outstanding Cardiology Resources from Williams & Wilkins

Heart Disease Diagnosis and Therapy: A Practical Approach

M. Gabriel Khan, MD, Eric J. Topol, MD, and Sanjeev Saksena, MD

Here is the perfect choice for board review, updated with current information. Clinically focused and problem-oriented, this small handbook provides the basics of cardiology in a concise format. The authors concentrate on pathophysiology, the foundation for effective therapy, and common cardiologic problems with an emphasis on practical pharmacologic management.

1996/680 pages/148 illustrations/0-683-04614-4

The Pharmacologic Management of Heart Disease

Joel Kupersmith, MD, and Prakash Deedwania, MD

Readers will find information on cardiac drugs in all categories, with a focus on management strategies for both normal and special situations. It covers important basic concepts of patient management, pharmacokinetics, and methods for evaluating drugs, along with management categories in the most important clinical areas: cardiac arrhythmias, ischemic heart disease, congestive heart failure, and anti-clotting and lipid lowering drugs.

1996/608 pages/105 illustrations/0-683-04796-5

Pearls & Pitfalls in Electrocardiography
Second Edition

Henry J.L. Marriott, MD, FACP, FACC

There are a number of electrocardiography books available, but none with the authority of Dr. Marriott, the acknowledged master of electrocardiography. His techniques, developed over years of clinical experience, have brought the art of interpreting electrocardiograms to a new level, and this text brings together a treasury of diagnostic gems.

1997/176 pages/20 illustrations/0-683-30170-5

Preview these texts for a full month. If you're not completely satisfied, return them at no further obligation (US and Canada only).

Phone orders accepted 24 hours a day, 7 days a week (US only).

From the US call: 1-800-638-0672
From Canada call: 1-800-665-1148
From outside the US and Canada call 410-528-4223
From the UK and Europe call 44 (171) 543-4800
From Southeast Asia call (852) 2610-2339

INTERNET

E-mail: custserv@wwilkins.com
Home page: http://www.wwilkins.com

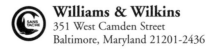 **Williams & Wilkins**
351 West Camden Street
Baltimore, Maryland 21201-2436